50 Imaging Studies Every Doctor Should Know

50 STUDIES EVERY DOCTOR SHOULD KNOW

Published and Forthcoming Books in the *50 Studies Every Doctor Should Know* Series

50 Studies Every Doctor Should Know: The Key Studies That Form the Foundation of Evidence Based Medicine, Revised Edition
Michael E. Hochman

50 Studies Every Internist Should Know
Kristopher Swiger, Joshua R. Thomas, Michael E. Hochman, and Steven D. Hochman

50 Studies Every Neurologist Should Know
David Y. Hwang and David M. Greer

50 Studies Every Surgeon Should Know
SreyRam Kuy, Rachel J. Kwon, and Miguel Burch

50 Studies Every Pediatrician Should Know
Ashaunta T. Anderson, Nina L. Shapiro, Stephen C. Aronoff, Jeremiah Davis, and Michael Levy

50 Imaging Studies Every Doctor Should Know
Christoph I. Lee

50 Studies Every Anesthesiologist Should Know
Anita Gupta

50 Studies Every Intensivist Should Know
Edward Bittner

50 Studies Every Psychiatrist Should Know
Vinod Srihari, Ish Bhalla, and Rajesh Tampi

50 Imaging Studies Every Doctor Should Know

EDITED BY

CHRISTOPH I. LEE, MD, MSHS

Associate Professor, Radiology
Adjunct Associate Professor, Health Services
University of Washington
Seattle, Washington

IMAGE AND CHAPTER EDITOR

JOSEPH S. FOTOS, MD

Assistant Professor, Radiology
Penn State Milton S. Hershey Medical Center
Hershey, Pennsylvania

SERIES EDITOR

MICHAEL E. HOCHMAN, MD, MPH

Assistant Professor, Medicine
Director, Gehr Family Center for Implementation Science
USC Keck School of Medicine
Los Angeles, California

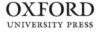

OXFORD
UNIVERSITY PRESS

Oxford University Press is a department of the University of Oxford. It furthers
the University's objective of excellence in research, scholarship, and education
by publishing worldwide. Oxford is a registered trade mark of Oxford University
Press in the UK and certain other countries.

Published in the United States of America by Oxford University Press
198 Madison Avenue, New York, NY 10016, United States of America.

Library of Congress Cataloging-in-Publication Data
Names: Lee, Christoph I., editor. | Fotos, Joseph S., editor.
Title: 50 imaging studies every doctor should know / edited by Christoph I. Lee ; image and chapter editor,
Joseph S. Fotos.
Other titles: Fifty imaging studies every doctor should know | 50 studies every doctor should know (Series)
Description: Oxford ; New York : Oxford University Press, 2017 | Series: 50 studies every doctor should
know | Includes bibliographical references and index.
Identifiers: LCCN 2016002868| ISBN 9780190223700 (alk. paper) | ISBN 9780190223724 (e-book) |
ISBN 9780190223731 (online)
Subjects: | MESH: Diagnostic Imaging—methods | Evidence-Based Medicine | Clinical Trials as Topic
Classification: LCC RC78.7.D53 | NLM WN 180 | DDC 616.07/54—dc23 LC record available at
http://lccn.loc.gov/2016002868

9 8 7 6 5 4 3 2 1

Printed by WebCom, Inc., Canada

For Monique, Elsa, and Carson

.

CONTENTS

SECTION 4 Abdominal and Pelvic Pain

PREFACE

This book was written as part of the *50 Studies Every Doctor Should Know* series, with the goal of familiarizing clinicians, medical trainees, and even interested patients with the key studies that form the foundation of evidence-based medical imaging. For almost every physician specialty, imaging examinations play a central role in the screening, diagnosis, and treatment management of diseases. These examinations are becoming more nuanced with technological advances, bringing even greater potential to lead to improved patient outcomes. However, many of these examinations also have unforeseen downsides, including increased health care costs and unnecessary downstream interventions.

The appropriate use of medical imaging requires a baseline understanding of the literature we use to decide whether or not a specific imaging study would be helpful in a specific clinical scenario. For the physician trying to make diagnoses in practice or on the wards, understanding the medical literature regarding imaging may feel both impractical and at times irrelevant. After all, guidelines from professional societies specify best practices in a digestible format. Is that not sufficient, particularly in a field like radiology?

The trouble is that clinical decision making is often nuanced and current guidelines are not exhaustive. For example, recent guidelines recommend routine screening mammograms in women 50–74 years of age. But do these recommendations apply to younger women with a strong family history of breast cancer? What about women who are very anxious about the disease but who do not fall within this age range? And what about for a frail woman in her 60s with numerous comorbidities? Key studies on screening mammography—summarized in this book—provide important insights that enable informed decisions in these gray areas where guidelines may not apply.

Some may argue that evidence-based practices may be less important in the field of radiology, which is often one step removed from direct patient care. To the contrary, evidence is particularly relevant when ordering imaging examinations for diagnostic purposes. First, proper treatment depends on an accurate diagnosis, and therefore it is essential that the proper test be ordered. Second, imaging tests may trigger a "cascade" of follow-up testing if the initial results are equivocal. Thus, it is critical that clinicians are parsimonious in selecting imaging examinations to avoid unnecessary tests and interventions. Finally, as you will learn in the section dedicated to radiation exposure, many imaging tests result in substantial exposure to ionizing radiation, which can be harmful. Using an evidence-based approach with imaging is important not only for obtaining the proper diagnosis but also to avoid inadvertent harm.

In this volume, we have attempted to identify key studies from the radiology literature and to present them in an accessible format. A small handful of the studies we selected come directly from the original edition of *50 Studies Every Doctor Should Know* but most are new to this edition. We begin each study summary by identifying the clinical question being addressed; we then summarize the main findings and methodological strengths and weaknesses. We conclude each summary by highlighting the central message and the implications for clinical practice. We also provide a clinical case at the end of each chapter, which gives you an opportunity to apply the findings in a real-life situation.

Although the study summaries in this volume focus on the field of radiology, we have written the book for a general medical audience. After all, it is nonradiologists who order most imaging examinations, and thus clinicians in all fields must be familiar with the evidence behind what they are ordering. Thus, only studies relevant to a broad range of clinicians are included.

You may wonder how we selected the studies included here. Based on feedback from the original edition of *50 Studies Every Doctor Should Know*, we used a rigorous selection process in which we surveyed experts in the field of internal medicine, and we used their input to develop our list. Even despite our efforts to use a systematic process to select studies, we suspect that some will disagree with our selections. Still, we believe the studies we describe cover a wide array of topics in medical imaging. As examples, we have included a meta-analysis of screening trials for carotid artery stenosis that supports guidelines against routine screening for this condition; the PIOPED II Trial, which demonstrated that computed tomography is a reliable method for screening for pulmonary embolism; and a study evaluating the Ottawa predictive rules that define when imaging is indicated for patients with ankle injuries. As always, we are happy to receive feedback and suggestions for future editions of this book.

Finally, we hope that you will finish this book not only with a strong understanding of the key studies in the field of radiology but also with a framework for reviewing clinical studies and applying the results to practice. We hope this will enable physicians and patients alike to make more thoughtful and informed decisions when ordering medical imaging examinations.

Happy reading!

Michael E. Hochman, MD, MPH, Series Editor,
50 Studies Every Doctor Should Know

Christoph I. Lee, MD, MSHS, Author,
50 Imaging Studies Every Doctor Should Know

ACKNOWLEDGMENTS

I would like to thank Dr. Michael Hochman, the series editor, for the opportunity to write this book and for allowing me to borrow several chapters from his original book in this series, *50 Studies Every Doctor Should Know*. As my former office mate and enduring friend, Dr. Hochman continues to be an inspiring figure in my professional life. I owe a debt of gratitude to Dr. Joseph Fotos for serving as a chapter text editor and for providing almost all of the excellent imaging examples found throughout the book. Andrea Knobloch and Rebecca Suzan at Oxford University Press have been extremely supportive, and simplified the logistics for this work. I also thank the several anonymous expert reviewers commissioned by Oxford who helped select the list of included studies.

I've been fortunate to have many mentors help guide me to successfully get to where I am today as a physician-scientist. I give special thanks to Drs. Howard Forman, Terry Desser, Carol Mangione, Norman Beauchamp, Connie Lehman, Jerry Jarvik, Janie Lee, Joann Elmore, and Scott Ramsey for their generosity and sage advice. I credit having the time and encouragement to write this book to my wife and best friend, Monique Mogensen, and my amazing family, including John, Jay, Bettina, Elena, Carson, and Elsa Lee.

Finally, I would like to thank the authors of the studies included in this book that I have listed hereafter. These authors graciously took the time to review the scientific summaries for accuracy. I am extremely appreciative of their assistance. Importantly, the views expressed in this book do not represent those of the authors acknowledged next, nor is the overall accuracy of information a reflection of their reviews; any mistakes remain my own.

Christoph Lee, MD, MSHS

- David R. Anderson, MD
- Wendy A. Berg, MD, PhD
- Enrico Bernardi, MD, PhD
- Sarah D. Berry, MD, MPH

- Rebecca Smith-Bindman, MD
- Michael N. Brant-Zawadzki, MD
- Suzanne M. Cadarette, PhD
- Martin Englund, MD, PhD
- Abdelilah el Barzouhi, MD
- Reza Fazel, MD, MSc
- Mieke Kriege, PhD
- Jerome R. Hoffmann, MD
- Udo Hoffman, MD, MPH
- Jeffrey G. Jarvik, MD, MPH
- Chelsea S. Kidwell, MD
- Harry J. de Koning, MD, PhD
- Nathan Kuppermann, MD, MPH
- C. Daniel Johnson, MD
- Daniel E. Jonas, MD, MPH
- Kyoung Ho Lee, MD
- Constance D. Lehman, MD, PhD
- Harold I. Litt, MD, PhD
- Paul J. Nederkoorn, MD, PhD
- Heidi D. Nelson, MD, MPH
- Jeffrey J. Perry, MD, MSc
- Perry J. Pickhardt, MD
- Etta D. Pisano, MD
- Paul D. Stein, MD
- Ian G. Stiell, MD, MSc
- Frans J. Th. Wackers, MD, PhD

ABOUT THE AUTHOR

Dr. Christoph Lee is a board-certified radiologist who earned his BA cum laude from Princeton University, his MD cum laude from Yale University, and his MS in health policy and management research from UCLA. He completed his radiology residency at Stanford University and a health policy fellowship as a Robert Wood Johnson Foundation Clinical Scholar. He joined the University of Washington School of Medicine as an assistant professor in 2012, and was promoted to associate professor in 2015. He holds additional faculty appointments at the Fred Hutchinson Cancer Research Center, the University of Washington School of Public Health, the Pacific Northwest Evidence-Based Practice Center, and RAND Health.

Dr. Lee is the lead editor and author of five textbooks spanning the basic sciences, evidence-based medicine, and medical imaging, distributed both nationally and internationally. He has obtained extramural research grants from major funding organizations including the National Institutes of Health (NIH), American Cancer Society, and Agency for Healthcare Research and Quality. Dr. Lee has authored more than 50 peer-reviewed journal articles, and currently serves on the editorial boards of the *American Journal of Roentgenology* and the *Journal of the American College of Radiology*. He is considered a national thought leader in imaging-related policy and health services research.

SECTION 1

Headache

Computed Tomography for Minor Head Injury

The New Orleans Criteria

CHRISTOPH I. LEE

> All patients with positive [CT] scans had at least one of . . . seven find-
> ings, resulting in a sensitivity of 100 percent . . . [and] a negative pre-
> dictive value of 100% [for detecting acute traumatic intracranial lesions
> following minor head trauma] . . .
>
> —HAYDEL ET AL.[1]

Research Question: When is a head computed tomography (CT) scan unnecessary to rule out an acute traumatic intracranial lesion for minor head injuries?

Funding: None declared.

Year Study Began: 1997

Year Study Published: 2000

Study Location: Single large inner-city level 1 trauma center.

Who Was Studied: Patients with loss of consciousness or amnesia after a traumatic event, at least 3 years of age, who presented within 24 hours after injury,

and who had both normal Glasgow Coma Scale scores (15 out of 15) and neurologic examinations at presentation.

Who Was Excluded: Patients who declined CT or who had concurrent injuries that precluded CT.

How Many Patients: 520 patients for first phase; 909 patients for second phase

Study Overview: This was a two-phase study. The first phase was to record clinical findings in consecutive patients presenting with minor head trauma, including demographic data, symptoms, and physical exam findings. Recursive partitioning (a statistical technique that creates a decision tree) was then used to derive a set of criteria to identify patients who had positive head CT findings (hematoma, hemorrhage, cerebral contusion, or depressed skull fracture). The second phase of the study involved prospectively evaluating the criteria's ability to predict a positive CT scan in a separate cohort of consecutive patients.

Study Protocol: Both the phase I and phase II study questionnaires were completed before the CT scan and included data regarding patient age, presence/absence of headache, vomiting, alcohol/drug intoxication, short-term memory loss, posttraumatic seizure, history of coagulopathy, and evidence of physical trauma above the clavicles.

Follow-Up: Patients were followed until discharge from the Emergency Department or hospital.

Endpoints: Sensitivity, specificity, and negative predictive value of the determined criteria.

RESULTS

- A total of 6.9% of phase I patients (36/520) and 6.3% (57/909) of phase II patients had positive CT scans (Figure 1.1).
- All patients with positive CT scans had at least 1 of 7 findings for both study phases:
  — headache
  — vomiting
  — age > 60 years
  — drug or alcohol intoxication
  — short-term memory deficit

— physical evidence of trauma above the clavicles
— seizure

- The 7 findings combined were associated with a sensitivity of 100% ([95%, 100%], 95% CI), negative predictive value of 100% ([99%, 100%], 95% CI), and specificity of 24% ([22%, 28%], 95% CI) for positive head CT scan findings (see Table 1.1).

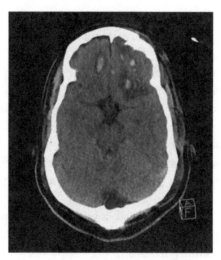

Figure 1.1 Axial noncontrast head CT with bifrontal hemorrhagic contusions secondary to blunt force head trauma. Note the associated cerebral edema.

Table 1.1. THE TRIAL'S KEY FINDINGS

Findings	Sensitivity	Specificity	Reduction in CT Use[a]
Short-term memory deficit, intoxication, trauma	94%	34%	31%
Short-term memory deficit, intoxication, trauma, age > 60 years, seizure	97%	31%	28%
Short-term memory deficit, intoxication, trauma, age > 60 years, seizure, headache, vomiting	100%	24%	22%

[a] Percent reduction in number of CT scans that would have resulted if criteria had been followed.

Criticisms and Limitations: Previous studies have suggested an association between presence of coagulopathy at presentation and a positive CT scan.[2,3] However, patients with coagulopathy were underrepresented in this study and this criterion could not be evaluated. Patients were not followed after discharge, so data are unavailable on delayed complications of minor head injuries. There have been reports of patients with initial negative CT scans subsequently found to have a traumatic lesion detected on follow-up CT.[4]

Other Relevant Studies and Information:

- A follow-up study evaluating the clinical decision rule (aka the New Orleans Criteria) in a pediatric population (N = 175, aged 5–17 years) with major mechanisms of injury resulting in minor head injury found that the presence of at least 1 of 6 clinical variables (headache, emesis, intoxication, seizure, short-term memory deficits, and physical evidence of trauma above the clavicles) was significantly associated with a positive CT scan ($P < 0.05$) and 100% sensitivity ([73%, 100%], 95% CI).[5]
- The Canadian Head CT rule was developed from a prospective cohort of patients seen at 10 large hospitals (N = 3,121) and consists of 5 high-risk factors (Glasgow Coma Scale score < 15 within 2 hours, suspected open skull fracture, any sign of basal skull fracture, vomiting > 2 episodes, or age > 65 years). These factors had 100% sensitivity ([92%, 100%], 95% CI) for positive CT scans, and would require only 32% of patients to undergo head CT.[6]
- External validation of both the New Orleans Criteria and the Canadian Head CT rule for patients with minor head injury was performed in a prospective multicenter trial in the Netherlands (N = 3,181). This study found that the Canadian Head CT rule has a lower sensitivity than the New Orleans Criteria for positive CT scans (83.4%–87.2% vs. 97.7%–99.4%, respectively).[7]
- American College of Radiology (ACR) Appropriateness Criteria for minor closed head injury (Glasgow Coma Scale ≥ 13 without neurologic deficit) rates a head CT scan without contrast as 7 out of 9 (usually appropriate).[8]

Summary and Implications: Head CT scans for patients with minor head injury can be safely limited to those presenting with at least 1 of 7 specific clinical findings: headache, vomiting, age >60 years, drug or alcohol intoxication, short-term memory deficit, physical evidence of trauma above the clavicles, and seizure. Application of the New Orleans Criteria could result in a 22% reduction in CT scan use, representing a substantial reduction in wasted health care resources and ionizing radiation exposure.

CLINICAL CASE: CT FOR MINOR HEAD INJURY

Case History:
You are evaluating a 16-year-old male brought to the emergency department directly after his involvement in a motor vehicle accident. The patient was the driver of the vehicle, and he experienced a brief loss of consciousness after his head hit the steering wheel just before the air bag deployed. His Glasgow Coma Scale score is 15 of 15 and he does not have any neurologic deficits on examination. He denies headache, nausea, vomiting, seizure, and memory deficits. On physical exam, he exhibits neck stiffness, as well as abrasions and burns involving his neck and forehead, likely from impact and airbag deployment. Based on the New Orleans Criteria, should you order a head CT for this patient?

Suggested Answer:
Based on the results of this study, ordering a head CT scan is indicated for this patient. The New Orleans Criteria apply to all patients >3 years of age with normal Glasgow Coma Scale scores (15 out of 15) and neurologic examinations at presentation. This patient does show evidence of physical trauma above the level of the clavicles, 1 of the 7 criteria associated with an acute traumatic intracranial lesion.

References

1. Haydel MJ, Preston CA, Mills TJ, et al. Indications for computed tomography in patients with minor head injury. *N Engl J Med*. 2000;343(2):100–105.
2. Stein SC, Young GS, Talucci RC, et al. Delayed brain injury after head trauma: significance of coagulopathy. *Neurosurgery*. 1992;30(2):160–165.
3. Gomez PA, Lobato RD, Ortega JM, et al. Mild head injury: differences in prognosis among patients with a Glasgow Coma Scale score of 13 to 15 and analysis of factors associated with abnormal CT findings. *Br J Neurosurg*. 1996;10(5):453–460.
4. Di Rocco A, Ellis SJ, Landes C. Delayed epidural hematoma. *Neuroradiology*. 1991;33(3):253–254.
5. Haydel MJ, Shembekar AD. Prediction of intracranial injury in children aged five years and older with loss of consciousness after minor head injury due to nontrivial mechanisms. *Ann Emerg Med*. 2003;42(4):507–514.

6. Stiell IG, Wells GA, Vandemheen K, et al. The Canadian CT Head Rule for pa-
    tients with minor head injury. *Lancet*. 2001;357(9266):1391–1396.
7. Smits M, Dippel DW, de Haan GG, et al. External validation of the Canadian CT
    Head Rule and the New Orleans Criteria for CT scanning in patients with minor
    head injury. *JAMA*. 2005;294(12):1519–1525.
8. American College of Radiology. ACR appropriateness criteria: head trauma.
    http://www.acr.org/~/media/C94E6287904E4D1CB185A7A63D1C0A37.pdf.
    Accessed December 13, 2014.

2

Identifying Children with Low-Risk Head Injuries Who Do Not Require Computed Tomography

MICHAEL E. HOCHMAN

[We] derived and validated highly accurate prediction rules for children at very low risk of [clinically important traumatic brain injuries] for whom CT scans should typically be avoided. Application of these rules could limit CT use, protecting children from unnecessary radiation risks.

—KUPPERMANN ET AL.[1]

Research Question: Is it possible to develop clinical prediction rules for identifying children at very low risk for clinically important traumatic brain injuries (ciTBIs) who do not require computed tomography (CT) scans for evaluation?

Funding: The Pediatric Emergency Care Applied Research Network (PECARN), a federally funded organization supported by the United States Health Resources and Services Administration.

Year Study Began: 2004

Year Study Published: 2009

Study Location: 25 emergency departments in the United States.

Who Was Studied: Children <18 years presenting to emergency departments within 24 hours of blunt traumatic head injuries.

Who Was Excluded: Children with "trivial" injuries such as ground-level falls without signs or symptoms of head injuries aside from scalp lacerations or abrasions, as well as children with penetrating trauma, brain tumors, and "pre-existing neurological disorders." In addition, children with ventricular shunts, bleeding disorders, and Glasgow Coma Scale (GCS) scores <14 were excluded from this analysis.

How Many Patients: 42,412

Study Overview: Prospective cohort study. In the derivation phase, binary recursive partitioning was used to derive a set of criteria with the goal of maximizing the negative predictive value and sensitivity of prediction rules. In the validation phase, performances of the rules were evaluated in similar, respective age cohorts.

Derivation of Prediction Rules: Emergency department physicians interviewed and examined a sample of children with head trauma (the derivation sample) to collect information about each child's history and physical examination findings. This information was collected prior to head imaging (if imaging was performed). The patient information was then correlated with patient outcomes (i.e., whether or not patients were ultimately found to have ciTBIs) in order to develop prediction rules for assessing brain injury risk.

Validation of Prediction Rules: The prediction rules were then applied to a separate sample of children (the validation sample) presenting with blunt head trauma to assess how well the rules forecasted whether or not these children would ultimately be diagnosed with ciTBIs.

Determination of Patient Outcomes: Research coordinators determined which children were ultimately diagnosed with ciTBIs by reviewing the medical records of all children admitted to the hospital. In addition, research coordinators conducted telephone interviews with the guardians of all children discharged from the emergency department to identify any children with missed injuries.

ciTBIs (see Figure 2.1) were defined as those resulting in:

- death from traumatic brain injury,
- neurosurgery,
- intubation for >24 hours, or
- hospital admission for ≥2 nights "associated with traumatic brain injury on CT."

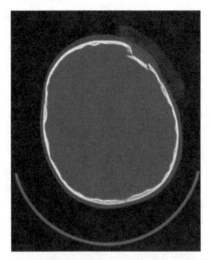

Figure 2.1 Axial noncontrast head CT image with depressed fracture of the left frontal bone secondary to blunt force head trauma.

The researchers did not classify "brief intubations" and single-night admissions for "minor CT findings" as ciTBIs because these outcomes do not typically represent clinically important injuries that must be identified; that is, patient outcomes would generally be unchanged if these injuries were never diagnosed.

RESULTS

- Table 2.1 lists the 6 predictive features for ciTBI identified using data from the derivation sample; the strongest predictors of ciTBI in both age groups were an abnormality in mental status or clinical evidence of a skull fracture.
- Table 2.2 divides children into 3 risk categories (low, medium, and high) using the predictive features.
- In the validation sample, 2 children, both older than 2 years, who did not exhibit any of the 6 predictive features, were ultimately found

to have ciTBIs. Both of these children were injured during sport-related activities, neither wore helmets, both had moderate headaches, and both had large frontal scalp hematomas; neither required neurosurgery.

Table 2.1. PREDICTORS OF CLINICALLY IMPORTANT TRAUMATIC BRAIN INJURIES

Children <2 Years
- Altered Mental Status[a]
- Palpable or Possibly Palpable Skull Fracture
- Occipital, Parietal, or Temporal Scalp Hematoma
- Loss of Consciousness ≥5 Seconds
- Severe Mechanism of Injury[b]
- Child Not Acting Normally According to Parents

Children ≥2 Years
- Altered Mental Status[a]
- Clinical Signs of Basilar Skull Fracture[c]
- Loss of Consciousness
- Vomiting
- Severe Mechanism of Injury[b]
- Severe Headache

[a] Defined as a Glasgow Coma Scale score of 14 or one of the following: agitation, somnolence, repetitive questioning, or a slow response to verbal communication.
[b] Defined as motor vehicle crash with patient ejection, death of another passenger, or rollover; pedestrian or bicyclist without helmet struck by motorized vehicle; falls >5 feet for children ≥2 years or >3 feet for those <2 years; or head struck by high-impact object.
[c] For example: retro-auricular bruising (Battle's sign), periorbital bruising (raccoon eyes), hematotympanum, or cerebral spinal fluid otorrhea or rhinorrhea.

Table 2.2. PROBABILITY OF CLINICALLY IMPORTANT TRAUMATIC BRAIN INJURIES BASED ON THE PRESENCE OF PREDICTIVE FEATURES FOR CHILDREN ≥2 YEARS[a]

Risk Category	Percentage of Children in This Category	Probability of ciTBI
Altered Mental Status or Evidence of a Basilar Skull Fracture	14.0%	4.3%
Any of the Four Predictive Features Other Than Altered Mental Status or Basilar Skull Fracture	27.7%	0.9%
None of the 6 Predictive Features	58.3%	<0.05%

[a] The numbers are similar for children <2 years except that the predictive features are different (see Table 2.1). For children <2 years, the highest risk categories are "Altered Mental Status" and "Palpable or Possibly Palpable Skull Fracture."

Criticisms and Limitations: Emergency departments were carefully selected for participation in this study. In real-world practice, clinicians—particularly those with less experience caring for children—may not be able to safely and effectively follow these prediction rules.

Because children change considerably between early infancy and 2 years of age, perhaps the prediction rule for this age group should be further stratified (e.g., a different rule for children <1 year and children 1–2 years).

Other Relevant Studies and Information:

- A follow-up analysis involving children in this study demonstrated that children who were observed in the emergency department for a period of time before a decision was made about obtaining a CT scan were less likely to receive a CT scan.[2]
- The PECARN prediction rules developed as part of this study have successfully been implemented in other settings.[3]
- Some studies have suggested that there may be as many as 1 case of lethal cancer due to radiation for every 1,000–5,000 head CT scans in children.[4]
- Several other prediction rules for determining when CT scans are indicated in children with head trauma have also been developed[5]; however, the rules developed in the PECARN study appear to be the best.[6]

Summary and Implications: This study derived and validated prediction rules that can accurately identify children at very low risk for ciTBI. The authors suggest that one way these rules could be applied is as follows:

- Children with none of the 6 predictive features are at very low risk (<0.05%) for ciTBI and typically do not require CT scans.
- Children with either of the 2 highest risk features—altered mental status or evidence of a skull fracture—are at high risk (approximately 4%) for ciTBI and should receive CT scans.
- Children with any of the 4 predictive features other than altered mental status or evidence of a skull fracture have an intermediate risk for ciTBI of approximately 0.9% and the decision about whether or not to obtain a CT should be individualized based on other factors, such as the clinician's judgment, the number of predictive features present, serial evaluations of the patient over time, and the family's preferences.

CLINICAL CASE: DETERMINING WHETHER OR NOT TO OBTAIN A HEAD CT

Case History:

An 18-month-old boy is brought to the emergency department by his parents after he fell off his parent's bed. The bed is approximately 3–4 feet off the ground, and he landed on the side of his head. The boy cried for several minutes after the fall, but he has been acting normally since. He did not lose consciousness after the fall.

On examination, he has a small abrasion over his right cheek, and he has tenderness to palpation over parts of the right parietal region of his scalp. He does not have any scalp hematomas or palpable skull fractures. His neurologic examination is normal.

Based on the results of this study, should you order a CT scan to evaluate this boy for a traumatic brain injury?

Suggested Answer:

The boy in this vignette has 1 of the 6 predictive features for a ciTBI for children <2 years: he had a severe mechanism of injury (fall from a height >3 feet). Based on this study, his risk for a ciTBI is approximately 0.9% (a more precise follow-up analysis estimates the risk for children <2 with a severe mechanism of injury but no other predictive features at 0.3%[7]). The authors of this study recommend that for children in this risk category, the decision about whether or not to obtain a head CT should be individualized based on the clinician's judgment and the family's preference.

As this boy's doctor, you might explain to his parents that the risk of brain injury is low. If you order a head CT scan, there is a small chance that you would detect an important abnormality, but most likely you would not. In addition, the radiation from the CT scan could be harmful. Thus, it would be reasonable either to proceed with the CT scan or to monitor the patient closely and only order a CT scan if the boy's condition worsens. You should engage the parents to determine the approach with which they are most comfortable.

References

1. Kuppermann N, Holmes JF, Dayan PS, et al. Identification of children at very low risk of clinically important brain injuries after head trauma: a prospective cohort study. *Lancet.* 2009;374:1160–1170.

2. Nigrovic LE, Schunk JE, Foerster A, et al. The effect of observation on cranial computed tomography utilization for children after blunt head trauma. *Pediatrics*. 2011;127(6):1067–1073.

3. Bressan S, Romanato S, Mion T, Zanconato S, Da Dalt L. Implementation of adapted PECARN decision rule for children with minor head injury in the pediatric emergency department. *Acad Emerg Med*. 2012;19(7):801.

4. Brenner DJ, Hall EJ. Computed tomography—an increasing source of radiation exposure. *N Engl J Med*. 2007;357:2277–2284.

5. Maguire JL, Boutis K, Uleryk EM, Laupacis A, Parkin PC. Should a head-injured child receive a head CT scan? A systematic review of clinical prediction rules. *Pediatrics*. 2009;124(1):e145.

6. Pickering A, Harnan S, Fitzgerald P, Pandor A, Goodacre S. Clinical decision rules for children with minor head injury: a systematic review. *Arch Dis Child*. 2011;96(5):414–421.

7. Nigrovic LE, Lee LK, Hoyle J, et al. Prevalence of clinically important traumatic brain injuries in children with minor blunt head trauma and isolated severe injury mechanisms. *Arch Pediatr Adolesc Med*. 2011;166(4):356–361.

3

Rule Out Subarachnoid Hemorrhage for Headache

The Ottawa Subarachnoid Hemorrhage Rule

CHRISTOPH I. LEE

> This rule may help to standardize which patients with acute headache require investigations and . . . decrease the relatively high rate of missed subarachnoid hemorrhages.
>
> —PERRY ET AL.[1]

Research Question: Can clinical decision rules accurately and reliably identify patients with acute headache requiring investigations to rule out subarachnoid hemorrhage (SAH)?

Funding: Canadian Institutes for Health Research, Ontario Ministry of Health, Vancouver Coastal Health Research Institute.

Year Study Began: 2006

Year Study Published: 2013

Study Location: Ten university-affiliated Canadian tertiary care emergency departments.

Who Was Studied: Consecutive adults (≥16 years) with an acute headache peaking within 1 hour and no neurologic deficits (Glasgow Coma Scale score of 15 of 15), no trauma (no fall or direct head trauma in previous 7 days), and presenting within 14 days of headache onset.

Who Was Excluded: Patients with 3 or more recurrent headaches of same intensity and character as presenting headache over period > 6 months; transferred from another hospital with confirmed subarachnoid hemorrhage, returning for reassessment of same headache already evaluated by CT and lumbar puncture; papilledema on funduscopic exam; new focal neurologic deficit; previous diagnosis of cerebral aneurysm, subarachnoid hemorrhage, brain tumor, or hydrocephalus.

How Many Patients: 2,131

Study Overview: Multicenter prospective cohort study.

Study Protocol: Physicians completed patient data forms (recording 19 clinical findings from prior derivation study) prior to imaging or lumbar puncture being completed. Diagnosis of subarachnoid hemorrhage was established a priori by consensus of 5 emergency physicians and 1 neurosurgeon. Refinement of decision rules was assessed using multivariate recursive partitioning.

Follow-Up: Telephone follow-up at 1 and 6 months after emergency department assessment and review of medical records and provincial coroner's office to identify patients who developed subarachnoid hemorrhage.

Endpoints: Accuracy, reliability, and refinement of clinical decision rules to rule out subarachnoid hemorrhage (subarachnoid blood on CT scan, xanthochromia in CSF, or RBCs in final tube of CSF, with positive angiography findings).

RESULTS

- 6.2% (132/2,131) of enrolled patients had subarachnoid hemorrhage.
- The final Ottawa SAH Rule had 100% (95% CI, 97.2%–100%) sensitivity and 15.3% (95% CI, 13.8%–16.9%) specificity for identifying subarachnoid hemorrhage, and included the following patient characteristics:
  — age ≥ 40 years
  — neck pain or stiffness
  — witnessed loss of consciousness
  — onset during exertion
  — thunderclap headache (instantly peaking pain)
  — limited neck flexion on examination.
- Bootstrap analysis (1,000 replications) for the Ottawa SAH Rule using the previous phase 1 derivation data set combined with the

new validation cohort found that the sensitivity for subarachnoid hemorrhage was 100% (95% CI, 98.6%–100%) and the specificity was 17.8% (95% CI, 16.6%–19.1%) (Table 3.1).

Table 3.1. THE TRIAL'S KEY FINDINGS

Candidate Decision Rule	Sensitivity[a]	Specificity[a]	Negative Predictive Value %
Rule 1: Investigate if ≥ 1 high-risk findings present: age ≥ 40 years, neck pain or stiffness, witnessed loss of consciousness, onset during exertion	98.5% (94.6%–99.6%)	27.6% (25.7%–29.6%)	99.6%
Rule 2: Investigate if ≥ 1 high-risk findings present: age ≥ 45 years, witnessed loss of consciousness, vomiting, diastolic blood pressure ≥ 100 mm Hg	95.5% (90.4%–97.9%)	30.6% (28.6%–32.6%)	99.0%
Rule 3: Investigate if ≥ 1 high-risk findings present: age 45–55 years, neck pain or stiffness, arrival by ambulance, systolic blood pressure ≥ 160 mm Hg	97.0% (92.5%–98.8%)	35.6% (33.6%–37.7%)	99.4%
Ottawa SAH Rule: Investigate if ≥ 1 high-risk findings present: all rule 1 characteristics plus thunderclap headache and limited neck flexion on exam	100.0% (97.2%–100.0%)	15.3% (13.8%–16.9%)	100.0%

[a] The 95% confidence interval is in parentheses.

Criticisms and Limitations: The inclusion criteria allowed patients with non-thunderclap headaches to be enrolled, diluting the acuity of headache onset; however, this was done by design to capture patients with less sudden SAH. There was also no gold standard definition for subarachnoid hemorrhage, with diagnosis determined by consensus. The final, derived clinical decision rule requires additional further evaluation in implementation studies.

Other Relevant Studies and Information:

- The three original candidate clinical decision rules evaluated in this study were prospectively derived in a previous cohort of 1,999 patients presenting with acute nontraumatic headache.[2]
- The Ottawa SAH Rule is only for identifying patients with subarachnoid hemorrhage and is not a rule for all acute headaches Thus, if a patient presents with a headache and isolated cranial nerve palsy, angiography may be indicated to evaluate for aneurysm at risk for acute rupture.[3]
- The American College of Emergency Medicine provides a "level B recommendation" (strategy reflecting moderate clinical certainty) for an emergent head CT for patients presenting with new sudden-onset severe headache.[4]
- American College of Radiology Appropriateness Criteria for sudden onset of severe headache ("worst headache of life" or "thunderclap headache") rate a head CT scan without contrast as 9 out of 9 (usually appropriate).[5]

Summary and Implications: The Ottawa SAH Rule has high sensitivity and high negative predictive value for identifying subarachnoid hemorrhage among patients presenting to the emergency department with acute nontraumatic headache that reached maximal intensity within 1 hour and with normal neurologic examinations (Figure 3.1).

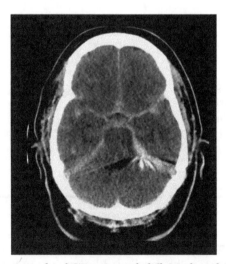

Figure 3.1 Axial noncontrast head CT image with diffuse subarachnoid hemorrhage in all basilar cisterns. This was secondary to recurrent bleed from previously clipped left posterior communicating artery aneurysm (note the partially visualized streak artifact).

CLINICAL CASE: RULE OUT SAH FOR ACUTE HEADACHE

Case History:

A 38-year-old male is visiting the emergency department due to an acute, severe headache that began 4 hours prior to his arrival. The patient's Glasgow Coma Scale score is 15, and physical exam demonstrates no limited neck flexion. The patient reports no neck pain or stiffness, loss of consciousness, thunderclap headache, or headache onset during exertion. He does have neurofibromatosis type I and an unruptured cerebral aneurysm, but no other medical conditions. Based on your history and physical, should you order a head CT to rule out subarachnoid hemorrhage?

Suggested Answer:

Even though the patient does not meet any of the criteria of the Ottawa SAH Rule, a noncontrast head CT scan is still indicated due to the patient's history of unruptured cerebral aneurysm. Patients with a history of cerebral aneurysm were excluded from this study.

References

1. Perry JJ, Stiell IG, Sivilotti ML, et al. Clinical decision rules to rule out subarachnoid hemorrhage for acute headache. *JAMA.* 2013;310(12):1248–1255.
2. Perry JJ, Stiell IG, Sivilotti ML, et al. High risk clinical characteristics for subarachnoid haemorrhage in patients with acute headache: prospective cohort study. *BMJ.* 2010;341:c5204.
3. Kissel JT, Burde RM, Klingele TG, et al. Pupil-sparing oculomotor palsies with internal carotid-posterior communicating artery aneurysms. *Ann Neurol.* 1983;13(2):149–154.
4. Edlow JA, Panagos PD, Godwin SA, et al. Clinical policy: critical issues in the evaluation and management of adult patients presenting to the emergency department with acute headache. *Ann Emerg Med.* 2008;52(4):407–436.
5. Douglas AC, Wippold FJ 2nd, Broderick DF, et al. ACR appropriateness criteria headache. *J Am Coll Radiol.* 2014;11(7):657–667.

4

MRI versus CT for Detecting Acute Intracerebral Hemorrhage in Stroke Patients

The Hemorrhage and Early MRI Evaluation (HEME) Study

CHRISTOPH I. LEE

> Due to its advantages in delineating ischemic pathophysiology, in combination with . . . equivalency to CT for detecting acute hemorrhage, MRI may be acceptable as the sole imaging technique for acute stroke . . .
> —KIDWELL ET AL.[1]

Research Question: Is MRI or CT more accurate for detecting acute intracranial hemorrhage in patients with acute focal stroke symptoms?

Funding: National Institute of Neurological Disorders and Stroke, American Heart Association, Heart & Stroke Foundation, and the Canadian Institutes for Health Research.

Year Study Began: 2000

Year Study Published: 2004

Study Location: Two stroke centers (UCLA Medical Center and Suburban Hospital, Bethesda, MD).

Who Was Studied: Patients presenting with focal stroke symptoms within 6 hours of onset (and definite last known well time).

Who Was Excluded: Patients with coma, pacemaker, or other contraindication to MRI; symptoms suggestive of subarachnoid hemorrhage; inability to obtain MRI within 6 hours of last known well time; initiation of thrombolytics, antithrombotics, and anticoagulants prior to completion of imaging studies; or cardiorespiratory instability precluding MRI.

How Many Patients: 200

Study Overview: Prospective multicenter cohort study of MRI versus CT for patients with acute stroke to establish that gradient recalled echo (GRE) MRI is sensitive to acute hemorrhage. An interim analysis found that MRI was detecting acute hemorrhages not seen on CT, and thus the study was stopped early in order to expedite the reporting of these important findings.

Study Protocol: All patients underwent 1.5-tesla MRI and then CT, with the goal of completing all imaging within 90 minutes of presentation to the emergency department. Both GRE and diffusion-weighted imaging had to be completed during the MRI to qualify for enrollment.

Follow-Up: Final hospital discharge diagnosis incorporated imaging, laboratory, pathologic, and clinical data. No follow-up after hospital discharge.

Endpoints: Primary endpoint was accuracy of MRI versus CT for detecting acute intracranial hemorrhage. Secondary endpoints were accuracy of MRI versus CT for any hemorrhage (acute or chronic) and for chronic hemorrhage. Outcomes were determined by consensus of four blind readers (two neuroradiologists and two stroke neurologists).

RESULTS

- Hemorrhage was accurately identified on MRI in all cases of acute intraparenchymal hematomas seen on CT.
- Acute hemorrhage was seen in 25 patients on both CT and MRI; 4 additional patients had acute hemorrhage seen as hypointensity on the GRE images within an ischemic field (seen on diffusion-weighted imaging) on the MRI.
- Interrater reliability based on the kappa statistic for paired observers of acute hemorrhage were 0.75–0.82 for MRI and 0.87–0.94 for CT.
- Chronic hemorrhage was seen on MRI but not on CT for 52 patients (Table 4.1).

Table 4.1. THE TRIAL'S KEY FINDINGS

Type of Hemorrhage	Positive CT	Negative CT	P Value
Any hemorrhage			
MRI +	28	43	.001
MRI −	1	128	
Chronic hemorrhage			
MRI +	0	52	<0.001
MRI −	0	148	

Criticisms and Limitations: In cases of small hemorrhages, acute and chronic hemorrhage may not be easily differentiated on GRE images alone, and a non-contrast head CT may be needed to determine hemorrhage age. Interreader reliability was better for CT than MRI; thus, institutions choosing to use MRI and not CT for evaluating acute stroke patients should provide a comprehensive educational program for physicians interpreting the MRI studies.

Other Relevant Studies and Information:

- Detecting intracranial hemorrhage is critical since it is a contraindication for use of thrombolytics. GRE pulse sequences can detect the paramagnetic effects of deoxyhemoglobin and methemoglobin (hyperacute hemorrhage) that may escape detection on CT[2–4].
- The B5 Hemorrhage Study performed by the German Stroke Competence Network evaluated the accuracy of MRI versus CT for differentiating acute intracerebral hematoma from acute ischemic stroke with patients randomized to MRI or CT first.[5] The prospective multicenter trial found that MRI with GRE images can rule out intracranial hemorrhage alone and demonstrate underlying pathology in hyperacute stroke.
- ACR Appropriateness Criteria for cerebrovascular disease and clinically suspected parenchymal hemorrhage rates a head CT scan without contrast as 9 out of 9 (usually appropriate) and head MRI as 6 out of 9 (may be appropriate).[6]
- The American Heart Association recommends MRI over CT for patients within 3 hours of onset of symptoms if the imaging does not delay the timely administration of intravenous thrombolytics.[7]

Summary and Implications: MRI is as accurate as CT for detecting acute hemorrhage in suspected stroke and is more accurate than CT for detecting chronic intracerebral hemorrhage (Figure 4.1).

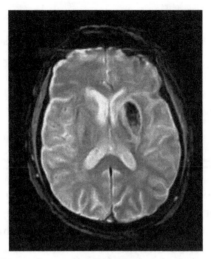

Figure 4.1 Axial gradient echo image of the brain with a large area of signal dropout representing a left basal ganglia hemorrhagic stroke.

CLINICAL CASE: MRI VERSUS CT FOR DETECTING ACUTE HEMORRHAGE

Case History:
A 56-year-old woman presents to your stroke center with facial droop and unilateral extremity weakness of 1-hour duration. You would like to provide antithrombolytic therapy, but are concerned about intracerebral hemorrhage. The stroke center has an on-site CT scanner as well as a 1.5 Tesla MRI scanner with echo-planar imaging capabilities and a standardized 10-minute multisequence imaging protocol. What imaging test should you preferentially order?

Suggested Answer:
Based on the HEME study and the B5 Hemorrhage Study, a brain MRI may be able to better identify intracranial hemorrhage and potentially identify the underlying pathology for this hyperacute stroke patient compared to a head CT. With rapid MRI imaging available on site with experienced stroke physicians who can interpret the study, a brain MRI is likely to provide more information than a noncontrast head CT scan and would be the preferable test.

References

1. Kidwell CS, Chalela JA, Saver JL, et al. Comparison of MRI and CT for detection of acute intracerebral hemorrhage. *JAMA*. 2004;292(15):1823–1830.
2. Patel MR, Edelman RR, Warach S. Detection of hyperacute primary intraparenchymal hemorrhage by magnetic resonance imaging. *Stroke* 1996;27(12):2321–2324.
3. Schellinger PD, Jansen O, Fiebach JB, et al. A standardized MRI stroke protocol: comparison with CT in hyperacute intracerebral hemorrhage. *Stroke*. 1999;30(4):765–768.
4. Atlas SW, Thulborn KR. MR detection of hyperacute parenchymal hemorrhage of the brain. *AJNR Am J Neuroradiol*. 1998;19(8):1471–1477.
5. Fiebach JB, Schellinger PD, Gass A, et al. Stroke magnetic resonance imaging is accurate in hyperacute intracerebral hemorrhage: a multicenter study on the validity of stroke imaging. *Stroke*. 2004;35(2):502–506.
6. DeLaPaz RL, Wippold FJ2nd, Cornelius RS, et al. ACR appropriateness criteria on cerebrovascular disease. *J Am Coll Radiol* 2011;8(8):532–538.
7. Latchaw RE, Alberts MJ, Lev MH, et al. Recommendations for imaging of acute ischemic stroke: a scientific statement from the American Heart Association. *Stroke* 2009;40(11):3646–3678.

5

Quantitative CT Score in Predicting Outcome of Hyperacute Stroke

The Alberta Stroke Programme Early CT Score (ASPECTS)

CHRISTOPH I. LEE

> We have shown that a systematic approach to quantification of early CT ischemic change can improve the identification of cerebral ischemia and is of prognostic value even before treatment is administered.
> —BARBER ET AL.[1]

Research Question: Can a quantitative score on baseline head CT for hyperacute stroke identify patients unlikely to recover despite thrombolytic therapy?

Funding: Alberta Stroke Programme.

Year Study Began: 1996

Year Study Published: 2000

Study Location: Two North American teaching hospitals.

Who Was Studied: Patients with symptoms suggestive of acute anterior-circulation ischemic stroke and who had a clearly defined time of onset, a deficit measurable on the National Institutes of Health Stroke Scale (NIHSS) by

≥4 points 24 hours after onset of stroke, a baseline CT scan showing no intra-cranial hemorrhage, and treatment within 3 hours of onset with intravenous alteplase.

Who Was Excluded: Patients with ischemia on head CT too extensive to treat with alteplase; patients treated with intravenous alteplase but identified clin-ically to have posterior circulation ischemia; and patients treated outside the established National Institute of Neurological Disorders and Stroke (NINDS) protocol.

How Many Patients: 156

Study Overview: All enrolled patients had a baseline CT scan and NIHSS score recorded by a stroke neurologist. A repeat NIHSS score was recorded before the 24-hour follow-up CT scan. The baseline CT scan was assessed with knowledge of the side affected but without knowledge of baseline imaging re-sults, NIHSS scores, or clinical outcomes by a panel of 3 stroke neurologists and 3 neuroradiologists. Outcome measures were scored on the modified Rankin Scale at 3 months (independence 0–2, dependence 3–5, and death), and symp-tomatic intracerebral hemorrhage. Predictive performance of the ASPECTS score was compared to the predictive performance of NIHSS scores of ≤15 (less severe) and ≥15 (more severe), as well as ischemia involving ≤ one-third of the middle cerebral artery (MCA) territory (less severe) and ≥ one-third of the MCA territory (more severe, less benefit from thrombolytic therapy).

Study Intervention: The ASPECTS 10-point quantitative CT scan score re-quires segmental assessment of the MCA territory with 1 point subtracted from the initial score of 10 if there is evidence of early ischemic change (e.g., focal swelling or parenchymal hypoattenuation) in a specific topographic region (caudate, putamen, internal capsule, insular cortex, M1–M6 vascular territo-ries). The score is calculated from two standard axial CT slices (one at level of thalamus and basal ganglia and one rostral to ganglionic structures). A score of 10 indicates a normal CT scan and a score of 0 indicates diffuse MCA-territory ischemia.

Follow-Up: Three-month outcomes assessment by stroke neurologist or stroke nurse blinded from all imaging and clinical notes.

Endpoints: Sensitivity and specificity for predicting symptomatic intrace-rebral hemorrhage and 3-month functional outcome after administration of alteplase.

RESULTS

- 117 of 156 (75%) of patients had early ischemic changes identified on their baseline head CT and 141 of 156 (90%) had ischemic changes on their 24-hour follow-up CT scan.
- ASPECTS scores were correlated inversely with stroke severity on the NIHSS ($r = -0.56$, $P < 0.001$).
- An ASPECTS score of ≤7 reliably predicted worse functional outcome at 3 months (discrimination between independence versus dependence or death) and higher risk of intracerebral hemorrhage (see Tables 5.1 and 5.2).

Table 5.1. THE TRIAL'S FUNCTIONAL OUTCOME FINDINGS

Test Measure	3-Month Functional Outcome		Sensitivity	Specificity
	Independent	Dependent or Dead		
ASPECTS Score				
>7 (n = 65)	71	18	0.78	0.96
≤7 (n = 89)	3	62		
NIHSS				
≤15 (n = 81)	56	25	0.69	0.76
>15 (n = 73)	18	55		
MCA Rule				
≤1/3 territory (n = 89)	67	22	0.73	0.91
>1/3 territory (n = 65)	7	58		

Table 5.2. THE TRIAL'S INTRACEREBRAL HEMORRHAGE FINDINGS

Test Measure	Symptomatic Hemorrhage Outcome		Sensitivity	Specificity
	Yes	No		
ASPECTS Score				
>7 (n = 91)	1	90	0.90	0.62
≤7 (n = 65)	9	56		
NIHSS				
≤15 (n = 81)	6	75	0.40	0.62
>15 (n = 73)	4	69		
MCA Rule				
≤1/3 territory (n = 91)	1	90	0.90	0.62
>1/3 territory (n = 65)	9	56		

Criticisms and Limitations: The ASPECTS scoring system is limited to the MCA territory of the brain, making scoring of watershed infarcts difficult on noncontrast head CT. Incorrect ASPECTS scoring may result in the setting of significant subcortical and age-related periventricular white matter changes or poor scan quality such as motion artifacts or patient tilt. In facilities where advanced imaging capabilities exist, diffusion-weighted imaging MRI or CT imaging with perfusion sequences may provide more optimal information regarding early ischemic changes.[2,3]

Other Relevant Studies and Information:

- The NIHSS is a serial measure of neurologic deficit with a 42-point scale that quantifies neurologic deficits in 11 different categories.[4] It reliably detects changes in neurologic deficit in acute stroke patients, and at least a 4-point deficit was required for inclusion in this study.
- Thrombolysis using intravenous recombinant tissue plasminogen activator (alteplase) within 3 hours of symptom onset may improve clinical outcomes in acute stroke patients, but at increased risk of symptomatic intracerebral hemorrhage.[5]
- The European Cooperative Acute Stroke Study (ECASS) highlighted the importance of early ischemic changes on CT for predicting benefits of using immediate thrombolysis, with patients most likely to benefit if CT ischemia involves < one-third of the MCA territory (Figure 5.1).[6,7]

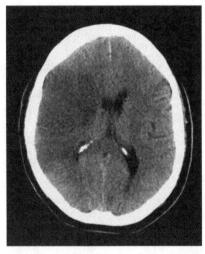

Figure 5.1 Axial noncontrast head CT image with a large area of hypodensity within the right MCA territory, representing a large right MCA ischemic stroke.

- The American Heart Association recommends MRI (with diffusion-weighted imaging and gradient-recalled echo sequences) over CT for patients within 3 hours of onset of symptoms if the imaging does not delay the timely administration of intravenous thrombolytics.[3] However, CT remains the most accessible imaging technology in the acute stroke setting.

Summary and Implications: The ASPECTS CT score may provide an objective, simple method for helping predict which acute stroke patients are unlikely to recover despite immediate thrombolytic therapy.

CLINICAL CASE: PREDICTING ACUTE STROKE OUTCOMES ON BASELINE CT SCAN

Case History:

A 56-year-old male presents to the emergency department with signs and symptoms of acute stroke, including hemiparesis, beginning 1 hour prior to arrival. You order a baseline CT scan that shows no intracranial hemorrhage. However, evaluation of two axial CT slices at the level of the basal ganglia and just rostral to the basal ganglia shows a focal area of cortical swelling of the left insular cortex and a focal area of hypoattenuation in the left internal capsule. As the consulting stroke neurologist, how would you weigh the risks of symptomatic ischemic hemorrhagic transformation versus functional improvement after treatment?

Suggested Answer:

Based on this study, this patient has an ASPECTS score of 8, and the functional benefits 3-months posttreatment are likely to outweigh the risks of hemorrhagic transformation. Indeed, in an acute stroke patient with an ASPECTS score >7, the rate of symptomatic intracerebral hemorrhage is about 1%, which is comparable to the frequency of symptomatic ischemic hemorrhagic transformation in the placebo group of the NINDS trial.[5]

References

1. Barber PA, Demchuk AM, Zhang J, et al. Validity and reliability of a quantitative computed tomography score in predicting outcome of hyperacute stroke before thrombolytic therapy. ASPECTS Study Group. Alberta Stroke Programme Early CT Score. *Lancet.* 2000;355(9216):1670–1674.

2. Albers GW, Lansberg MG, Norbash AM, et al. Yield of diffusion-weighted MRI for detection of potentially relevant findings in stroke patients. *Neurology.* 2000;54(8):1562–1567.

3. Latchaw RE, Alberts MJ, Lev MH, et al. Recommendations for imaging of acute ischemic stroke: a scientific statement from the American Heart Association. *Stroke* 2009;40(11):3646–3678.

4. Lyden P, Brott T, Tilley B, et al. Improved reliability of the NIH Stroke Scale using video training. NINDS TPA Stroke Study Group. *Stroke.* 1994;25(11):2220–2226.

5. Tissue plasminogen activator for acute ischemic stroke. The National Institute of Neurological Disorders and Stroke rt-PA Stroke Study Group. *N Engl J Med.* 1995;333(24):1581–1587.

6. Hacke W, Kaste M, Fieschi C, et al. Intravenous thrombolysis with recombinant tissue plasminogen activator for acute hemispheric stroke. The European Cooperative Acute Stroke Study (ECASS). *JAMA.* 1995;274(13):1017–1025.

7. Hacke W, Kaste M, Fieschi C, et al. Randomised double-blind placebo-controlled trial of thrombolytic therapy with intravenous alteplase in acute ischaemic stroke (ECASS II). Second European-Australasian Acute Stroke Study Investigators. *Lancet.* 1998;352(9136):1245–1251.

Imaging Selection and Endovascular Treatment for Ischemic Stroke

The Mechanical Retrieval and Recanalization of Stroke Clots Using Embolectomy (MR RESCUE) Trial

CHRISTOPH I. LEE

> Our findings do not support the efficacy of using CT or MRI to select patients for acute stroke management or the efficacy of mechanical embolectomy with first generation devices.
>
> —KIDWELL ET AL.[1]

Research Question: Can brain imaging identify patients most likely to benefit from therapies for acute ischemic stroke, including endovascular thrombectomy?

Funding: National Institute of Neurological Disorders and Stroke, with some study catheters and devices provided by Concentric Medical.

Year Study Began: 2004

Year Study Published: 2013

Study Location: 22 study sites in North America.

Who Was Studied: Patients aged 18–85 years, with National Institutes of Health Stroke Scale scores of 6–29 (on a scale of 0–42) who had large-vessel, anterior-circulation ischemic stroke presenting within 8 hours after onset of symptoms.

Who Was Excluded: Of the 127 patients who were eligible and underwent randomization, 9 were excluded (6 randomized to embolectomy and 3 randomized to standard care). Among patients randomized to embolectomy, 5 did not have a target lesion on vessel imaging and 1 had failed perfusion imaging. Among patients randomized to standard care, 2 did not have vessel imaging after tissue plasminogen activator (t-PA) use and 1 had failed perfusion imaging.

How Many Patients: 118

Study Overview: This phase 2b randomized controlled open-label (blinded outcome) trial assigned patients within 8 hours after onset of large-vessel, anterior-circulation strokes to standard care or mechanical embolectomy. All patients underwent pre-treatment multimodal CT or MRI of the brain. Randomization was stratified according to whether patients had favorable penumbral pattern (substantial salvageable tissue defined as predicted infarct core of ≤90 mL and predicted infarct tissue within at-risk region of ≤70%) or nonpenumbral pattern (small or absent salvageable tissue).

Study Intervention: Multimodal CT or MRI scans with perfusion sequences were performed at baseline. Embolectomy patients were treated with FDA-approved devices (MERCI Retriever and Penumbra System). For standard of care patients, intra-arterial t-PA at a dose of 14 mg or less was administered within 6 hours after symptom onset.

Follow-Up: CT or MRI perfusion imaging was performed at day 7. Functional outcomes were determined at day 90.

Endpoints: The primary functional outcomes were assessed using a 90-day modified Rankin Scale, ranging from 0 (no symptoms) to 6 (dead), with 0–2 classified as having a good functional outcome. The Thrombolysis in Cerebral Infarction (TICI) scale was used to assess successful revascularization (ranging from 0 for no perfusion to 3 for full perfusion).

RESULTS

- Across the study cohort, the rate of all-cause 90-day mortality was 21% and the rate of symptomatic intracerebral hemorrhage was 58%, with no significant difference across groups.
- Mean scores on the modified Rankin Scale did not differ between standard of care and embolectomy groups (3.9 vs. 3.9, $P = 0.99$).
- Outcomes for embolectomy were not any better than standard care, regardless of favorable penumbral pattern (mean scores = 3.9 vs. 3.4, $P = 0.23$) or a nonpenumbral pattern (mean scores = 4.0 vs. 4.4; $P = 0.32$).
- There were no significant differences in reperfusion or revascularization (TICI score = 2a–3) rates on 7-day imaging across groups; however, the final infarct volume was lower in patients with a favorable penumbra pattern regardless of treatment assignment (Table 6.1).

Table 6.1. THE TRIAL'S KEY FINDINGS

Outcome	Study Group				
	Embolectomy, Penumbra (n = 34)	Standard Care, Penumbra (n = 34)	Embolectomy, Nonpenumbral (n = 30)	Standard Care, Nonpenumbra (n = 20)	P Value[a]
Good outcome on 90-day modified Rankin Scale— n (%)	7 (21)	9 (26)	5 (17)	2 (10)	0.48
Death—n (%)	6 (18)	7 (21)	6 (20)	6 (30)	0.75
Symptomatic hemorrhage— n (%)	3 (9)	2 (6)	0	0	0.24
Reperfusion— n/total n (%)	16/28 (57)	14/27 (52)	7/19 (37)	6/12 (50)	0.59
Revascularization— n/total n (%)	20/30 (67)	25/27 (93)	20/26 (77)	14/18 (78)	0.13

[a] *P* values are for overall comparison across four groups; alpha level of significance was 0.05.

Criticisms and Limitations: Neutral results partly may have been due to low rate of substantial revascularization in the embolectomy group due to use of first-generation devices; newer-generation devices have had higher revascularization rates and better clinical outcomes than the MERCI Retriever.[2,3] The heterogeneity of imaging approaches (both MRI and CT used) may have contributed to neutral study results, as CT tended to show larger predicted core volumes than MRI. Patients with earlier time windows (<3 hours) and large-vessel occlusions and poor collateral vessels may benefit from recanalization, while a favorable penumbral pattern in later time windows may represent a biomarker for good outcomes due to better collateral flow and tolerance for occlusion.[4]

Other Relevant Studies and Information:

- The theory behind recanalization to reverse or minimize the deleterious effects of acute ischemic stroke is based on the hypothesis that brain tissue with reduced blood flow at risk of infarction (penumbra) can be salvaged if flow is restored in a timely manner.[5]
- The Diffusion and Perfusion Imaging Evaluation for Understanding Stroke Evolution (DEFUSE 2) study found that 46 of 78 (59%) patients with baseline MRI scans suggesting presence of salvageable tissue had reperfusion after endovascular treatment; however 12 of 21 (57%) patients without such findings on MRI also had reperfusion after endovascular treatment.[6] Target mismatch patient with early reperfusion had more favorable outcomes.
- The Local Versus Systemic Thrombolysis for Acute Ischemic Stroke (SYNTHESIS) trial randomly assigned 362 patients in Italy to either endovascular therapy or intravenous t-PA within 4.5 hours after symptom onset. The study found that endovascular therapy was not superior to standard treatment with intravenous t-PA based on survival free of disability at 3 months.[7]
- The Interventional Management of Stroke III (IMS III) randomized controlled trial, involving 656 patients, showed similar safety outcomes and no significant difference in functional independence with endovascular therapy after intravenous t-PA compared to intravenous t-PA alone.[8]
- For patients that are outside the window for intravenous t-PA but within the window for endovascular therapy (<8 hours since onset), the American College of Radiology, Society of NeuroInterventional Surgery, and American Society of Neuroradiology all recommend either multimodality CT (noncontrast head CT + CT angiography ± CT perfusion) or MRI (with at least diffusion-weighted imaging and gradient-recalled echo) ± MR angiography.[9]

Summary and Implications: A favorable penumbral pattern by CT or MRI imaging does not help identify patients who would benefit from endovascular therapy for acute stroke (Figures 6.1 and 6.2). Moreover, embolectomy is not superior to standard care with regard to clinical and imaging outcomes for acute ischemic stroke.

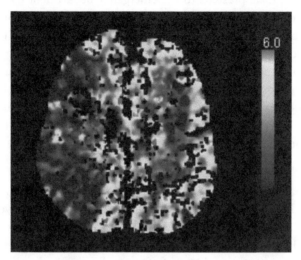

Figure 6.1 Axial CT perfusion cerebral blood volume image with significantly decreased blood volume within the right MCA territory, representing a large right MCA ischemic stroke.

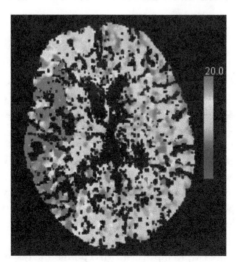

Figure 6.2 Axial CT perfusion time to peak image with significantly increased time to peak flow (conversely expressed as decreased blood flow) within the right MCA territory representing a large right MCA ischemic stroke.

CLINICAL CASE: ENDOVASCULAR TREATMENT BASED ON BRAIN IMAGING FINDINGS

Case History:

A 48-year-old male presents to the emergency department with signs and symptoms of acute ischemic stroke with symptom onset 3 hours prior to arrival. A noncontrast CT scan ordered by the triage nurse practitioner that showed no intracranial hemorrhage did show findings suggestive of a moderate-size left middle cerebral artery (MCA) infarct. The neurointerventional fellow would like to obtain an MRI with MR angiography and perfusion sequences to determine if endovascular therapy is warranted in this patient. Should you order this study given the patient's time window since symptom onset?

Suggested Answer:

Since the patient is still within the window for standard care with intravenous t-PA, this potentially life-saving therapy should not be delayed for more advanced imaging. The MR RESCUE study found no evidence that either CT or MRI findings to evaluate for imaging penumbra could help in determining which patients would benefit from endovascular therapy. Moreover, both the SYNTHESIS and IMS III trials did not show superiority of endovascular treatment over standard treatment among ischemic stroke patients.

References

1. Kidwell CS, Jahan R, Gornbein J, et al. A trial of imaging selection and endovascular treatment for ischemic stroke. *N Engl J Med.* 2013;368(10):914–923.
2. Nogueira RG, Lutsep HL, Gupta R, et al. Trevo versus Merci retrievers for thrombectomy revascularisation of large vessel occlusions in acute ischaemic stroke (TREVO 2): a randomised trial. *Lancet.* 2012;380(9849):1231–1240.
3. Saver JL, Jahan R, Levy EI, et al. Solitaire flow restoration device versus the Merci Retriever in patients with acute ischaemic stroke (SWIFT): a randomised, parallel-group, non-inferiority trial. *Lancet.* 2012;380(9849):1241–1249.
4. Shuaib A, Butcher K, Mohammad AA, et al. Collateral blood vessels in acute ischaemic stroke: a potential therapeutic target. *Lancet Neurol.* 2011;10(10):909–921.
5. Fisher M. Characterizing the target of acute stroke therapy. *Stroke.* 1997;28(4):866–872.
6. Lansberg MG, Straka M, Kemp S, et al. MRI profile and response to endovascular reperfusion after stroke (DEFUSE 2): a prospective cohort study. *Lancet Neurol.* 2012;11(10):860–867.

7. Ciccone A, Valvassori L, Nichelatti M, et al. Endovascular treatment for acute ischemic stroke. *N Engl J Med.* 2013;368(10):904–913.
8. Broderick JP, Palesch YY, Demchuk AM, et al. Endovascular therapy after intravenous t-PA versus t-PA alone for stroke. *N Engl J Med.* 2013;368(10):893–903.
9. Wintermark M, Sanelli PC, Albers GW, et al. Imaging recommendations for acute stroke and transient ischemic attack patients: A joint statement by the American Society of Neuroradiology, the American College of Radiology, and the Society of NeuroInterventional Surgery. *AJNR Am J Neuroradiol.* 2013;34(11):E117–E127.

7

Imaging Tests for Diagnosis of Carotid Artery Stenosis

CHRISTOPH I. LEE

... our results suggest that MRA [MR angiography] has a better discriminatory power compared with DUS [duplex ultrasound] in recognizing 70% to 99% stenosis ... For detecting occlusion of the carotid artery, both modalities are very accurate.

—NEDERKOORN ET AL.[1]

Research Question: Which imaging test is most accurate in diagnosing carotid artery stenosis?

Funding: The Dutch Ministry of Health, Welfare, and Sports, and the Netherlands Organization for Scientific Research.

Year Study Published: The individual studies were published between 1994 and 2001. This systematic review and meta-analysis was published in 2003.

Study Overview: This was a systematic review and meta-analysis of published data on the diagnostic value of duplex ultrasound (DUS), magnetic resonance angiography (MRA), and digital subtraction angiography (DSA) for identifying severe carotid artery stenosis.

Which Publications Were Included: A total of 63 publications were identified using an exhaustive search strategy. The systematic review and meta-analysis included results from 64 different patient series on DUS and 21 patient series on MRA.

Study Intervention: Inclusion of a study in the systematic review and meta-analysis required that MRA and/or DUS was used to estimate the severity of carotid artery stenosis and that DSA was used as the standard of reference.

Endpoints: All studies included in this systematic review required the absolute numbers of true positives, false negatives, true negatives, and false positives available or derivable for at least one degree of carotid artery stenosis. Pooled sensitivity and specificity of imaging tests were calculated from the available data. The pooled value of D (the natural logarithm of the diagnostic odds ratio) was calculated for each test. In addition, multivariable comparative modeling was performed to compare performance of imaging tests for detecting 70%–99% stenosis and occlusion.

RESULTS

- The pooled values of D were very similar across tests: 4.1 (95% CI, 3.5–4.8) for MRA and 4.0 (95% CI, 3.5–4.5) for DUS in diagnosing 70%–99% stenosis; 6.5 (95% CI, 5.7–7.4) for MRA and 6.5 (95% CI, 5.9–7.0) for DUS in diagnosing occlusion (Table 7.1).
- Upon multivariable modeling, verification bias and choice of cutoff for defining severe stenosis were associated with better DUS performance; for occlusion, the presence of verification bias (decision to perform reference standard test depends on results of the DUS test) and type of DUS scanner were significant predictors.
- The type and strength of MR scanner used was a significant predictor for MRA diagnostic performance in multivariate analysis for diagnosing 70%–99% stenosis.
- Multivariable modeling adjusting for significant predictors demonstrated that MRA had better discriminatory power than DUS for diagnosing 70%–99% stenosis from <70% stenosis (regression coefficient, 1.6; 95% CI, 0.37–2.77); however, there was no difference between MRA and DUS for differentiating occlusion from <100% stenosis (regression coefficient, 0.73; 95% CI –2.06 to 3.51).

Table 7.1. SUMMARY OF POOLED WEIGHTED SENSITIVITY AND SPECIFICITY

Degree of Carotid Artery Stenosis	Pooled Sensitivity % (95% CI)		Pooled Specificity % (95% CI)	
	MRA	DUS	MRA	DUS
70%–99% stenosis (versus <70% stenosis)	95 (92–97)	86 (84–89)	90 (86–93)	87 (84–90)
100% stenosis (versus <100% stenosis)	98 (94–100)	96 (94–98)	100 (99–100)	100 (99–100)

Criticisms and Limitations: The reference standard for this study was conventional angiography, which is itself limited by the number of projections on vessel lumens; the extent of plaque and plaque morphology associated with stenosed vessels are more readily appreciated on DUS and MRA.[2,3] Many studies were excluded from this analysis if absolute numbers of true positives, false negatives, true negatives, and/or false positives were not available or derivable. Since this meta-analysis, CT angiography (CTA) has been added to the other noninvasive tests (MRA and DUS) for presurgical evaluation of carotid stenosis.

Other Relevant Studies and Information:

- The North American Symptomatic Carotid Endarterectomy Trial (NASCET) and the European Carotid Surgery Trial (ECST) proved that carotid endarterectomy had mortality benefit for patients with severe (70-99%) symptomatic carotid artery stenosis.[4,5] Both trials used DSA as the standard of reference for selecting patients for surgery, which is associated with a relatively high risk of morbidity and mortality (1%–4%).[6]
- Later-generation MRA (either time of flight MRA or contrast enhanced MRA), CTA, and DUS have essentially replaced conventional angiography in the presurgical evaluation of carotid stenosis. A 2006 meta-analysis of 41 studies demonstrated high sensitivity and specificity for all three imaging exams for identifying 70%–99% stenosis in symptomatic patients, with marginally greater accuracy with MRA.[7]
- Some groups, including the Society of Radiologists in Ultrasound, suggest that a combination of DUS and MRA obviates the need

for DSA, particularly when the tests agree on the degree of
stenosis.[8,9]

• The American College of Cardiology, American Stroke Association,
  American Heart Association, American College of Radiology,
  and multiple other societies jointly recommend noninvasive DUS
  for initial diagnostic testing in patients with symptoms or signs of
  extracranial carotid artery disease, followed by MRA or CTA for
  patients with equivocal DUS or acute focal ischemic neurological
  symptoms.[10]

Summary and Implications: Both DUS and MRA are very accurate for detecting carotid artery occlusion; however, MRA is more accurate than DUS in
diagnosing 70%–99% carotid artery stenosis (Figure 7.1).

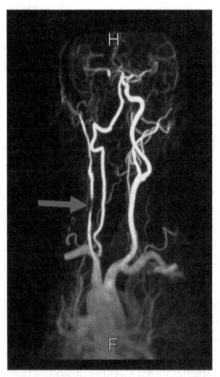

Figure 7.1 Coronal MRA image of the head and neck with a focal area of stenosis
within the right common carotid artery (arrow).

CLINICAL CASE: BEST IMAGING TEST FOR CAROTID ARTERY STENOSIS

Case History:

A 64-year-old male with a 40-pack-year smoking history, third-degree AV block with a pacemaker implanted, hypercholesterolemia, and type 2 diabetes presents to your primary care office complaining of intermittent headaches and intermittent left-sided weakness and tingling that resolves within minutes. Upon further questioning, he admits that he also experiences episodes of confusion and some blurry vision with the bouts of severe headaches. With concern about symptomatic carotid artery stenosis, which imaging study or studies should be ordered?

Suggested Answer:

Based on this systematic review and updated societal guidelines, noninvasive imaging with DUS and potentially CTA is the preferred exam(s) for presurgical evaluation and diagnosis of severe carotid artery stenosis. Given the patient's pacemaker, MRA would be contraindicated. DUS is highly accurate in determining stenosis >70%, and CTA can be considered to more fully characterize intraluminal plaque. Conventional angiography, associated with relatively higher morbidity and mortality, should be reserved for equivocal cases after noninvasive imaging.

References

1. Nederkoorn PJ, van der Graaf Y, Hunink MG. Duplex ultrasound and magnetic resonance angiography compared with digital subtraction angiography in carotid artery stenosis: a systematic review. *Stroke.* 2003;34(5):1324–1332.
2. Pan XM, Saloner D, Reilly LM, et al. Assessment of carotid artery stenosis by ultrasonography, conventional angiography, and magnetic resonance angiography: correlation with ex vivo measurement of plaque stenosis. *J Vasc Surg.* 1995;21(1):82–88; discussion 88–89.
3. Elgersma OE, Wust AF, Buijs PC, et al. Multidirectional depiction of internal carotid arterial stenosis: three-dimensional time-of-flight MR angiography versus rotational and conventional digital subtraction angiography. *Radiology.* 2000;216(2):511–516.
4. Barnett HJ, Taylor DW, Eliasziw M, et al. Benefit of carotid endarterectomy in patients with symptomatic moderate or severe stenosis. North American

Symptomatic Carotid Endarterectomy Trial Collaborators. *N Engl J Med.* 1998;339(20):1415–1425.

5. Randomised trial of endarterectomy for recently symptomatic carotid stenosis: final results of the MRC European Carotid Surgery Trial (ECST). *Lancet* 1998;351(9113):1379–1387.

6. Hankey GJ, Warlow CP, Molyneux AJ. Complications of cerebral angiography for patients with mild carotid territory ischaemia being considered for carotid endarterectomy. *J Neurol Neurosurg Psychiatry.* 1990;53(7):542–548.

7. Wardlaw JM, Chappell FM, Best JJ, et al. Non-invasive imaging compared with intra-arterial angiography in the diagnosis of symptomatic carotid stenosis: a meta-analysis. *Lancet.* 2006;367(9521):1503–1512.

8. Grant EG, Benson CB, Moneta GL, et al. Carotid artery stenosis: gray-scale and Doppler US diagnosis—Society of Radiologists in Ultrasound Consensus Conference. *Radiology.* 2003;229(2):340–346.

9. Turnipseed WD, Kennell TW, Turski PA, et al. Combined use of duplex imaging and magnetic resonance angiography for evaluation of patients with symptomatic ipsilateral high-grade carotid stenosis. *J Vasc Surg.* 1993;17(5):832–839; discussion 839–840.

10. Brott TG, Halperin JL, Abbara S, et al. 2011ASA/ACCF/AHA/AANN/AANS/ACR/ASNR/CNS/SAIP/SCAI/SIR/SNIS/SVM/SVS guideline on the management of patients with extracranial carotid and vertebral artery disease. A report of the American College of Cardiology Foundation/American Heart Association Task Force on Practice Guidelines, and the American Stroke Association, American Association of Neuroscience Nurses, American Association of Neurological Surgeons, American College of Radiology, American Society of Neuroradiology, Congress of Neurological Surgeons, Society of Atherosclerosis Imaging and Prevention, Society for Cardiovascular Angiography and Interventions, Society of Interventional Radiology, Society of NeuroInterventional Surgery, Society for Vascular Medicine, and Society for Vascular Surgery. *Circulation.* 2011;124(4):e54–e130.

8

Carotid Artery Stenosis Screening

CHRISTOPH I. LEE

> Reliability of ultrasonography is questionable because accuracy can vary considerably among laboratories. Its use in a low-prevalence population would result in many false-positives . . .
>
> —JONAS ET AL.[1]

Research Question: Should asymptomatic adults be screened for carotid artery stenosis (which accounts for approximately 10% of ischemic strokes)?

Funding: Agency for Healthcare Research and Quality.

Year Study Published: The results of individual studies published through March 2014 were included in the analysis. This systematic review was published in September 2014.

Study Locations: The included trials were conducted in multiple developed countries, mostly in North America and Europe.

Study Overview: This was a systematic review and meta-analysis of the existing literature performed for the US Preventive Services Task Force (USPSTF) to aid in determining their updated recommendations for population-based carotid artery stenosis screening.

Which Trials Were Included: 78 published articles that reported on 56 studies of good or fair quality were identified using an exhaustive search of MEDLINE, the Cochrane Library, EMBASE, and trial registries. The target patient population of each trial or study included was asymptomatic adults with carotid artery stenosis of potential clinical importance (defined as 60%–99% stenosis). Studies enrolling both symptomatic and asymptomatic patients were included if asymptomatic patients were analyzed separately.

Study Interventions: Screening with carotid DUS. Intervention for asymptomatic stenosis using carotid endarterectomy, carotid angioplasty and stenting, or medical therapy (e.g., aspirin, statins, antiplatelet medications).

Endpoints: Accuracy of imaging-based screening tests for identifying significant, but asymptomatic, carotid artery stenosis. Incremental benefits of intervention for asymptomatic stenosis. Risks of stroke or death and other harms due to intervention for asymptomatic stenosis.

RESULTS

- Duplex ultrasound has a sensitivity and specificity for detecting potentially clinically significant stenosis of 90%–98% and 88%–94%, respectively[2,3] (see Table 8.1 and Figure 8.1); however, accuracy varies widely across laboratories.
- Benefits of intervention after screening include a 5.5% (95% CI, 3.9%–7.0%) absolute reduction of nonperioperative strokes over approximately 5 years for carotid endarterectomy compared with medical therapy.
- No studies addressed anxiety among persons with false-positive results; however, potential harms associated with screening include unnecessary diagnostic workup, including risks associated with conventional angiography.

Table 8.1. SUMMARY OF DUPLEX ULTRASOUND ACCURACY

Degree of Carotid Artery Stenosis	Sensitivity % (95% CI)	Specificity % (95% CI)
≥50%	98% (97%–100%)	88% (76%–100%)
≥60%	94%*	92%*
≥70%	90% (84%–94%)	94% (88%–97%)

* No confidence interval was reported.

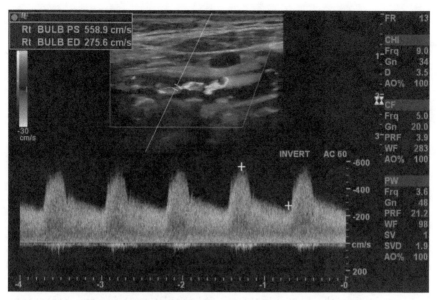

Figure 8.1 Sagittal Doppler image of the right carotid artery bulb with luminal narrowing, significantly increased velocity, and increased turbulence of flow consistent with severe stenosis.

- Harms associated with carotid endarterectomy for asymptomatic carotid artery stenosis include 30-day stroke rate of 2.4% (95% CI, 1.7%–3.1%), 30-day death rate of 3.3% (95% CI, 2.7%–3.9%), and smaller rates of cranial nerve damage, myocardial infarction, and postoperative hematoma.
- Compared with medical therapy patients (e.g., 325 mg aspirin therapy daily), intervention patients experienced a 1.9% (95% CI, 1.2%–2.6%) greater incidence of perioperative (30-day) stroke or death.

Criticisms and Limitations: Screening ultrasound accuracy is highly variable across laboratory settings, and is operator dependent. The medical therapies examined in trials were often not clearly defined or standardized, and many are now outdated. The benefits of interventions may have been overestimated (e.g., highly selected surgeons with low complication rates) while harms have been underreported and not reported.

Other Relevant Studies and Information:

- The ACAS (Asymptomatic Carotid Atherosclerosis Study), VACS (Veterans Affairs Cooperative Study), and the ACST (Asymptomatic Carotid Surgery Trial) collectively showed that asymptomatic carotid artery stenosis patients treated with endarterectomy had fewer perioperative strokes, deaths, or subsequent ipsilateral strokes than patients in medical therapy groups.[4–6]

- Using prevalence of significant carotid artery stenosis of 1% and ultrasound specificity of 92%, 940 true positives and 7,920 false positives would result from 100,000 screens. Even if positive ultrasound screens were followed by MR angiography (95% sensitivity, 90% specificity),[7] 792 false-positive results per 100,000 screened would undergo unnecessary intervention.
- Currently, the USPSTF recommends against screening for asymptomatic carotid artery stenosis in the general adult population.[8]

Summary and Implications: There is little evidence that the benefits of carotid endarterectomy, stenting, or intensification of medical therapy outweigh the risks among patients with asymptomatic carotid artery stenosis. The overall benefit of screening for asymptomatic carotid artery stenosis is limited by the low prevalence of the disease in the general population and known harms associated with downstream intervention.

CLINICAL CASE: SCREENING FOR CAROTID ARTERY STENOSIS

Case History:
A 64-year-old male patient presents to your primary care clinic with the desire to prevent strokes. He has a history of hypertension and hyperlipidemia well controlled on medical therapy, but recently had a brother who suffered a severe ischemic stroke. He has been reading articles online and specifically wants to discuss obtaining a screening duplex ultrasound to ensure that he does not need intervention for carotid artery stenosis. History and physical exam suggest no recent TIAs or other signs and symptoms suggestive of significant carotid artery stenosis. How would you counsel this patient?

Suggested Answer:
Currently, the USPSTF does not recommend routine screening for asymptomatic carotid artery stenosis in any patient population. You can begin by reviewing the patient's most recent laboratory results and reassuring him that his medication regimen is being effective in decreasing his hypertension and hyperlipidemia, known stroke risk factors. You can also explain to him that screening ultrasound, while widely offered, has not been shown to improve downstream patient outcomes and can lead to known harms of unnecessary interventions, including periprocedural strokes and death.

References

1. Jonas DE, Feltner C, Amick HR, et al. Screening for asymptomatic carotid artery stenosis: a systematic review and meta-analysis for the U.S. Preventive Services Task Force. *Ann Intern Med*. 2014;161(5):336–346.

2. Jahromi AS, Cina CS, Liu Y, et al. Sensitivity and specificity of color duplex ultrasound measurement in the estimation of internal carotid artery stenosis: a systematic review and meta-analysis. *J Vasc Surg*. 2005;41(6):962–972.

3. Wolff T, Guirguis-Blake J, Miller T, et al. Screening for carotid artery stenosis: an update of the evidence for the U.S. Preventive Services Task Force. *Ann Intern Med*. 2007;147(12):860–870.

4. Endarterectomy for asymptomatic carotid artery stenosis. Executive Committee for the Asymptomatic Carotid Atherosclerosis Study. *JAMA*. 1995;273(18):1421–1428.

5. Halliday A, Harrison M, Hayter E, et al. 10-year stroke prevention after successful carotid endarterectomy for asymptomatic stenosis (ACST-1): a multicentre randomised trial. *Lancet*. 2010;376(9746):1074–1084.

6. Hobson RW, 2nd, Weiss DG, Fields WS, et al. Efficacy of carotid endarterectomy for asymptomatic carotid stenosis. The Veterans Affairs Cooperative Study Group. *N Engl J Med*. 1993;328(4):221–227.

7. Nederkoorn PJ, van der Graaf Y, Hunink MG. Duplex ultrasound and magnetic resonance angiography compared with digital subtraction angiography in carotid artery stenosis: a systematic review. *Stroke*. 2003;34(5):1324–1332.

8. LeFevre ML. Screening for asymptomatic carotid artery stenosis: U.S. Preventive Services Task Force recommendation statement. *Ann Intern Med*. 2014;161(5):356–362.

Back Pain

9

Vertebroplasty for Osteoporotic Spinal Fractures

The Investigational Vertebroplasty Safety and Efficacy Trial (INVEST)

CHRISTOPH I. LEE

> ... at 1 month, clinical improvement in patients with painful osteoporotic vertebral fractures was similar among those treated with vertebroplasty and those treated with a simulated procedure.
>
> —KALLMES ET AL.[1]

Research Question: Does cement vertebroplasty decrease disability and pain for patients with osteoporotic vertebral body fractures?

Funding: National Institute of Arthritis and Musculoskeletal and Skin Diseases.

Year Study Began: 2004

Year Study Published: 2009

Study Location: Five medical centers in the United States, 5 medical centers in the United Kingdom, and 1 center in Australia with established vertebroplasty practices for osteoporotic fractures.

Who Was Studied: Adult patients age ≥50 years, diagnosis of 1–3 painful osteoporotic vertebral compression fractures between vertebral levels T4 and L5, inadequate pain relief by medical therapy, pain intensity score ≥3 (scale 0–10), and pain duration <1 year. For fractures of uncertain age, additional inclusion criteria of marrow edema on MRI or increased vertebral body uptake on nuclear medicine bone scan.

Who Was Excluded: Patients with neoplasm or suspicion of neoplasm in target vertebral body, substantial bony fragment retropulsion, active infection, concurrent hip fracture, uncontrollable bleeding diastheses, surgery within previous 60 days, no phone access, non-English speaking, or dementia.

How Many Patients: 131 patients were enrolled. Patients were randomized to either vertebroplasty (n = 68) or simulated procedure without cement (n = 63). Baseline characteristics between the two groups were similar.

Study Overview: Multicenter randomized controlled trial with intention-to-treat analysis.

Study Intervention: All practitioners were highly experienced with vertebroplasty. Using fluoroscopic guidance and with patients under conscious sedation, practitioners performed the same local anesthesia steps before patients were randomized to one of the two trial arms. Patients were allowed to cross over after 1 month if pain relief was inadequate.

Follow-Up: A vertebroplasty practitioner saw each patient in clinic 1 month postprocedure.

Endpoints: Disability score (modified Roland-Morris Disability [RMDQ] Questionnaire, scale 0–23, higher scores indicating greater disability) and average pain intensity rating during preceding 24 hours and at 1 month postprocedure (scale 0–10, higher scores indicating more severe pain).

RESULTS

- The mean RMDQ scores at 1 month postprocedure did not significantly differ between study groups (adjusted treatment effect 0.7, 95% CI: –1.3 to 2.8). The confidence interval excluded a treatment benefit of 3 points or more on the RMDQ scale, thus providing evidence against clinically meaningful treatment effects (Table 9.1).

- The mean pain intensity rating at 1 month postprocedure did not significantly differ between study groups (adjusted treatment effect 0.7, 95% CI: –0.3 to 1.7). The confidence interval excluded a benefit of 2 points or more.
- The two study groups had similar improvements in back-related disability and pain immediately after the procedure (3 days), and maintained improvements at 1 month postprocedure. There was a nonsignificant trend toward a higher rate of clinically meaningful improvement in pain in the vertebroplasty group than in the control group at 1 month (64% vs. 48%, $P = 0.06$).
- A single patient in each group had an adverse event. One patient in the vertebroplasty group had a thecal sac injury requiring hospitalization, and one patient in the control group had tachycardia and rigors of unknown origin requiring hospitalization.

Table 9.1. THE TRIAL'S KEY FINDINGS

Measure	Group (Mean ± SD)		P value[a]
	Vertebroplasty	Control	
RMDQ[b]			
At baseline	16.6 ± 3.8	17.5 ± 4.1	0.49
At 1 month	12.0 ± 6.3	13.0 ± 6.4	
Pain Intensity			
At baseline	6.9 ± 2.0	7.2 ± 1.8	0.19
At 1 month	3.9 ± 2.9	4.6 ± 3.0	

[a] P values from analysis of covariance models adjusted for study group assignment, baseline values of outcome measures, and study center; $P < 0.05$, statistically significant.
[b] Roland-Morris Disability Questionnaire.

Criticisms and Limitations: The study sample size was modified due to difficulty in patient recruitment. There was a higher crossover rate among patients in the control group versus the vertebroplasty group, which may be due to higher rates of unsatisfactory pain outcomes among control group patients not detected with this study's pain intensity measures. Since physicians and patients were reluctant to accept a longer period than 1 month to consider crossover, interpretation of outcomes after 1 month was complicated for between-group differences. Report of persistent back pain after vertebroplasty may be due to causes of pain other than from the osteoporotic fracture.

Other Relevant Studies and Information:

- Percutaneous vertebroplasty, involving injection of medical cement (polymethylmethacrylate) into the fractured vertebral body, remains a common procedure for routine therapy and pain relief for osteoporotic vertebral fractures (Figure 9.1).[2]
- Buchbinder et al performed a multicenter, randomized, double-blind, placebo-controlled trial in Australia where patients with 1–2 painful, unhealed osteoporotic vertebral fractures of <12 months' duration were assigned to vertebroplasty or a sham procedure.[3] They found no beneficial effect of vertebroplasty as compared with a sham procedure at 1 week or at 1, 3, or 6 months after intervention.
- The American Academy of Orthopaedic Surgeons (AAOS) Guidelines lists kyphoplasty as an option for neurologically intact patients with painful osteoporotic vertebral compression fractures, but note that the supporting evidence is weak.[4] The AAOS recommends against vertebroplasty for patients with an osteoporotic spinal compression fracture on imaging with correlating clinical signs and symptoms and who are neurologically intact.
- ACR Appropriateness Criteria for management of vertebral compression fractures recommends conservative management as

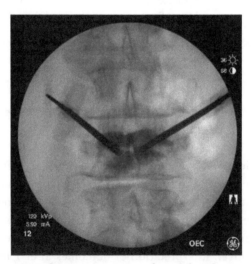

Figure 9.1 Intraoperative fluoroscopic image of a vertebroplasty procedure. The large-bore needles are inserted into the vertebral body via the pedicles bilaterally, followed by the administration of cement into the fracture cavity.

first-line therapy with vertebroplasty and kyphoplasty reserved for cases unresponsive to conservative management or progressing to neurological deficits.[5]

- The National Institute for Health and Clinical Excellence in the United Kingdom recommends vertebroplasty and kyphoplasty as possible treatment options for patients with painful osteoporotic vertebral compression fractures who do not respond to analgesics.[6]

Summary and Implications: For patients with pain from osteoporotic vertebral compression fractures of <1 year duration, patients undergoing vertebroplasty show similar improvements in back pain intensity, functional disability, and quality of life compared to patients undergoing a simulated vertebroplasty without cement injection at 1 month after intervention. Thus, factors aside from cement installation, such as a placebo effect, likely account for observed clinical improvements after vertebroplasty.

CLINICAL CASE: PAINFUL OSTEOPOROTIC SPINAL FRACTURE

Case History:

A 64-year-old female with osteoporosis and no major comorbidities visits your primary care clinic after having a lumbar spine MRI for persistent back pain performed a week prior. The radiologist reports a moderate upper lumbar spine vertebral compression fracture at the L2 level without retropulsion. She has been on calcitonin therapy along with nonsteroidal anti-inflammatories for pain relief. She reports 6 out of 10 pain with focal pain over the L2 vertebral body on physical exam. She is otherwise neurologically intact. She would like to inquire about preventing further compression with vertebroplasty.

Suggested Answer:

Based on this randomized controlled trial and societal guidelines, vertebroplasty is not recommended for painful osteoporotic compression fractures in patients who are neurologically intact. Conservative management should be the first-line therapy, including anti-osteoporotic medications (calcitonin), analgesics and nonsteroidal anti-inflammatory drugs, and physical therapy. Surgical intervention may be indicated in patients who develop neurological impairment (e.g., paresis, saddle anesthesia, bowel or bladder issues).

References

1. Kallmes DF, Comstock BA, Heagerty PJ, et al. A randomized trial of vertebroplasty for osteoporotic spinal factures. *N Engl J Med.* 2009; 361(6):569–579.

2. Buchbinder R, Golmohammadi K, Johnston RV, et al. Percutaneous vertebroplasty for osteoporotic vertebral compression fracture. *Cochrane Database Syst Rev.* 2015;4:CD006349. doi:10.1002/14651858.CD006349.pub2.

3. Buchbinder R, Osborne RH, Ebeling PR, et al. A randomized trial of vertebroplasty for painful osteoporotic vertebral fractures. *N Engl J Med.* 2009;361(6):557–568.

4. American Academy of Orthopaedic Surgeons. The treatment of symptomatic osteoporotic spinal compression fractures: guideline and evidence report. http://www.aaos.org/research/guidelines/SCFguideline.pdf. Published September 24, 2010. Accessed March 30, 2015.

5. McConnell CTJr, Wippold FJ2nd, Ray CEJr, et al. ACR appropriateness criteria management of vertebral compression fractures. *J Am Coll Radiol.* 2014;11(8):757–763.

6. National Institute for Health and Care Excellence. Percutaneous vertebroplasty and percutaneous balloon kyphoplasty for treating osteoporotic vertebral compression fractures. http://www.nice.org.uk/guidance/ta279. Published April 2013. Accessed March 30, 2015.

10

Cervical Spine Imaging in Blunt Trauma Patients

The National Emergency X-Radiography Utilization Study (NEXUS)

CHRISTOPH I. LEE

> ... this prospective, multicenter study confirms the validity of a decision instrument based on five clinical criteria for identifying, with a high degree of confidence, patients with blunt trauma who have an extremely low probability of having sustained injury to the cervical spine.
> —HOFFMAN ET AL.[1]

Research Question: Can a decision rule help avoid the need for cervical spine x-ray in cases of blunt trauma?

Funding: Agency for Healthcare Research and Quality.

Year Study Began: Not reported.

Year Study Published: 2000.

Study Location: 21 emergency departments (academic and community) across the United States.

Who Was Studied: Patients with blunt trauma who underwent cervical spine radiography (standard three views including cross-table lateral, anteroposterior, and open-mouth odontoid views).

Who Was Excluded: Patients with penetrating trauma, patients undergoing cervical spine imaging for reason other than trauma.

How Many Patients: 34,069

Study Overview: Prospective, multicenter, observational study.

Study Intervention: Decision instrument involving 5 criteria in order to classify a patient as having low probability of injury: no posterior midline cervical spine tenderness, no focal neurological deficit, normal level of alertness, no evidence of intoxication, and no clinically apparent pain elsewhere that might distract from cervical spine pain.

Follow-Up: Review of neurosurgical medical records and quality-assurance logs (but follow-up time period unspecified).

Endpoints: The sensitivity, specificity, negative predictive value, and positive predictive value of the decision instrument for predicting clinically significant cervical spine injury confirmed on radiography (Figure 10.1).

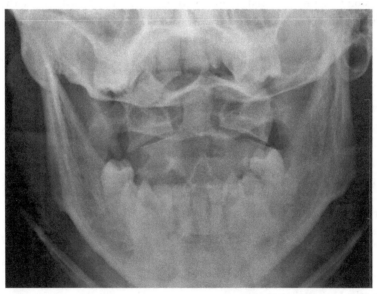

Figure 10.1 Type II odontoid fracture with slight right lateral displacement of the odontoid fracture fragment. Note the associated lateral displacement of the right lateral mass of C1.

RESULTS

- Of the 34,069 patients with imaging of the cervical spine for trauma, 818 (2.4%) had radiographically documented cervical spine injury.
- The decision instrument yielded a false-negative result in 8 of 818 patients with cervical spine injury, and 2 of these 8 patients were among the 518 with predefined clinically significant injury (CSI) (and only 1 of 2 required treatment).
- Use of all five criteria was necessary for the decision instrument to achieve 99.0% sensitivity, as some patients with CSIs only fulfilled one criterion (Table 10.1).
- According to the decision instrument classifications, 4,309 patients (12.6%) could have avoided radiographic evaluation, while 29,760 (87.4%) appropriately underwent cervical spine imaging.
- Using this decision instrument, the overall rate of missed cervical spine injuries would be less than 1 in 4,000 patients.

Table 10.1. CRITERIA PERFORMANCE IN RULING OUT C-SPINE TRAUMA

Characteristic	Value (%)	95% CI
All patients		
Sensitivity	99.0	(98.0–99.6)
NPV	99.8	(99.6–100)
Specificity	12.9	(12.8–13.0)
Patients with significant injury		
Sensitivity	99.6	(98.6–100)
NPV	99.9	(99.8–100)
Specificity	12.9	(12.8–13.0)

Criticisms and Limitations: Investigators chose not to explicitly define the individual criteria of the decision instrument, allowing variable interpretation by individual practitioners. This study was strictly observational, and some patients with cervical spine injury at study sites that met criteria but did not undergo radiography were not included in the study. With a specificity of 12.9%, there are concerns that the use of NEXUS criteria could actually increase overall use of radiography in some regions of the United States.

Other Relevant Studies and Information:

- The NEXUS criteria were validated among 2,943 geriatric patients, who are at increased risk of odontoid fracture and other CSIs after trauma. The NEXUS decision instrument for CSI in the geriatric group was 100% (95% CI, 97.1%–100%).[2]

- Another report focused on 3,065 pediatric trauma patients (age < 18 years), for whom the NEXUS criteria identified all CSIs (n = 30) (sensitivity = 100%; 95% CI: 87.8%–100.0%) and correctly designated 603 patients as low risk for CSI (NPV = 100%; 95% CI: 99.4%–100.0%).[3]
- The ACR Appropriateness Criteria concur with the NEXUS decision instrument in the case of suspected spine trauma in patients meeting the low-risk criteria.[4]

Summary and Implications: This set of five straightforward, logical diagnostic criteria approaches 100% sensitivity for identifying clinically important cervical spine injuries in patients with blunt trauma. Its widespread application could lead to both clinical and economic benefits by eliminating one-eighth of all cervical spine radiographs ordered for this patient population.

CLINICAL CASE: TRAUMA C-SPINE IMAGING

Case History:

A 13-year-old male patient is brought to the emergency department by his parents after a minor motor vehicle accident in which they were rear-ended. The patient denies any posterior midline cervical spine tenderness on examination, and has no focal neurological deficit. He exhibits a normal level of alertness, no signs of intoxication, and no clinically apparent pain elsewhere. His parents would like to get a battery of tests to make sure that nothing has been injured. Should you order a set of plain films to rule out cervical spine injury?

Suggested Answer:

The NEXUS study included all patients regardless of age. Thus, the decision rule would apply in the case of this 13 year-old who meets all five negative criteria. An additional analysis of the NEXUS criteria for 3,065 pediatric patients confirmed 100% sensitivity for CSI and 100% negative predictive value among the younger patient cohort. A standard three-view cervical spine radiograph examination therefore would not be of benefit in this case. You should reassure the parents that no imaging study is warranted and that the radiation and costs associated with cervical spine imaging would likely outweigh any potential benefit in this case.

References

1. Hoffman JR, Mower WR, Wolfson AB, Todd KH, Zucker MI; National Emergency X-Radiography Utilization Study Group. Validity of a set of clinical criteria to rule out injury to the cervical spine in patients with blunt trauma. *N Engl J Med*. 2000; 13:343(2)94–99.
2. Touger M, Gennis P, Nathanson N, et al. Validity of a decision rule to reduce cervical spine radiography in elderly patients with blunt trauma. *Ann Emerg Med*. 2002;40(3):287–293.
3. Viccellio P, Simon H, Pressman BD, Shah MN, Mower WR, Hoffman JR; NEXUS Group. A prospective multicenter study of cervical spin injury in children. *Pediatrics*. 2001;108(2):E20.
4. Daffner RH, Hackney DB. ACR Appropriateness Criteria on suspected spine trauma. *J Am Coll Radiol*. 2007;4(11):762–775.

11

Cervical Spine Imaging in Alert and Stable Trauma Patients

Validation of the Canadian C-Spine Rule

CHRISTOPH I. LEE

> ... we estimate that a 25% to 50% relative reduction in the use of C-spine radiography could be safely achieved.
>
> —STIELL ET AL.[1]

Research Question: Can a clinical decision rule allow physicians to be more selective in use of cervical spine imaging among alert and stable adult trauma patients?

Funding: Medical Research Council of Canada, Ontario Ministry of Health Emergency Health Services Committee, and the Canadian Institutes of Health Research.

Year Study Began: 1996

Year Study Published: 2001

Study Location: 10 large Canadian community and university hospitals.

Who Was Studied: Consecutive adult patients presenting to the emergency department after sustaining acute blunt trauma to the head or neck. Patients were included if they had neck pain from any mechanism of injury, or no neck pain but all of the following: some visible injury above the clavicles, had not been ambulatory, and had sustained a dangerous mechanism of injury (fall from an elevation ≥1 m or 5 stairs, axial load to the head, high-speed motor vehicle collision, roll over, ejection, bicycle collision, motorized vehicle collision). Patients also had to be alert (Glasgow Coma Scale [GCS] score of 15 out of 15) and stable (normal vital signs including systolic blood pressure > 90 mm Hg and respiratory rate between 10–24/minute).

Who Was Excluded: Patients <16 years old; did not meet inclusion criteria above; injury occurred >48 hours previously; penetrating trauma; acute paralysis; known vertebral disease (ankylosing spondylitis, rheumatoid arthritis, spinal stenosis, or previous cervical surgery); returned for reassessment of same injury; pregnant.

How Many Patients: 8,924

Study Overview: Prospective cohort study to collect clinical findings data; patients underwent cervical spine radiography (minimum of 3 views) at the discretion of the treating physician after the clinical assessment; logistic regression and chi-square recursive partitioning techniques to develop clinical decision rule.

Study Intervention: Physician evaluation of 25 standardized clinical variables (from the history, physical examination, and medical records) prior to cervical spine radiography.

Follow-Up: All enrolled patients who did not undergo cervical spine imaging underwent 14-day follow-up telephone interview administered by a registered nurse.

Endpoints: Clinically important cervical spine injury was defined as any fracture, dislocation, or ligamentous instability demonstrated by diagnostic imaging or 14-day proxy outcome measure administered by nurse over the phone. The sensitivity and specificity for the derived rule were calculated.

RESULTS

- Of the 8,924 patients, 151 (1.7%) were determined to have a clinically important cervical spine injury. An additional 28 (0.3%) of patients had clinically unimportant cervical spine injuries (e.g., isolated avulsion fracture of an osteophyte).

- The "Canadian C-Spine Rule" (CCR) asks 3 basic questions to determine whether or not cervical spine imaging is required for alert and stable trauma patients with concern for cervical spine imaging:
  1. Is there any high-risk factor present that mandates radiography (i.e., age ≥ 65 years, dangerous mechanism, or paresthesias in extremities)? If yes, then radiograph. If not, then ask the following:
  2. Is there any low-risk factor present that allows safe assessment of range of motion (i.e., simple rear-end motor vehicle collision, sitting position in emergency department, ambulatory at any time since injury, delayed onset of neck pain, or absence of midline cervical spine tenderness)? If not, then radiograph. If yes, then ask the following:
  3. Is the patient able to actively rotate his/her neck 45 degrees to the left and right? If yes, then no radiograph. If unable, then radiograph.
- The potential cervical spine radiography rate could be 58.2% in this cohort when using the decision rule, a relative reduction of 15.5% from the actual radiography rate of 68.9% (Table 11.1).
- Patients 65 years or older and those experiencing paresthesias were at considerable risk for cervical spine injury, and warrant radiography.

Table 11.1. THE TRIAL'S KEY FINDINGS

Decision Rule Performance Measure	Percentage	95% CI
Sensitivity	100	(98–100)
Specificity	42.5	(40–44)

Criticisms and Limitations: Not all eligible patients were enrolled in the study, opening up the possibility of selection bias. Not all study patients underwent cervical spine radiography (some had outcomes measured by a structured 14-day telephone-proxy outcome tool).

Other Relevant Studies and Information:

- A follow-up prospective cohort study in 9 Canadian emergency departments compared the CCR and the National Emergency X-Radiography Utilization Study (NEXUS) among 8,283 patients. The CCR was more sensitive than NEXUS criteria (99.4% vs. 90.7%, $P < 0.001$) and more specific than NEXUS criteria (45.1% vs. 36.8%) for identifying clinically important cervical-spine injuries.[2]

- The CCR was prospectively validated among Canadian nurses in emergency departments[3] and Canadian paramedics outside of the hospital setting,[4] and further validated via a matched-pair-cluster randomized trial.[5]
- The ACR Appropriateness Criteria concur with the CCR decision instrument in the case of suspected spine trauma in patients meeting the low-risk criteria.[6]
- In cases where cervical spine imaging is recommended by CCR or NEXUS criteria, CT of the cervical spine is now preferred over radiographs of the cervical spine.[7,8] CT also has a higher ACR appropriateness score than radiograph of the cervical spine.[6]

Summary and Implications: The Canadian C-Spine Rule may be able to identify a large group of alert and stable adult trauma patients for whom cervical spine imaging is unnecessary (Figure 11.1). It may also help to standardize the appropriate use of cervical spine imaging in the emergency department.

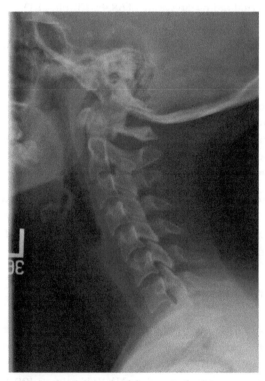

Figure 11.1 Normal lateral radiograph of the cervical spine.

CLINICAL CASE: C-SPINE TRAUMA IMAGING

Case History:

A 48-year-old female presents to the emergency department after a fall down a staircase and complaints of neck pain. She is alert (GCS score of 15 out of 15) with normal vital signs including a systolic blood pressure of 130 mm Hg and respiratory rate 16/minute. She denies any neurological symptoms or deficits. What further questions should you ask her during your history, and what will you examine physically in order to determine whether cervical spine imaging is required?

Suggested Answer:

Based on the Canadian C-Spine Rule, the patient has already fulfilled the first major criteria (there are no obvious high-risk factors demanding immediate imaging). On further questioning, you should determine if there are any low-risk factors present that would allow you to safely assess her neck's range of motion (i.e., if she is in a sitting position in the emergency department, delayed onset of neck pain, denied midline cervical tenderness). If not, then cervical spine imaging is warranted. If there is a low-risk factor present, then you may ask the patient to attempt to rotate her neck 45 degrees to the left and right. If she is able to do so, then no cervical spine imaging is warranted.

References

1. Stiell IG, Wells GA, Vandemheen KL, et al. The Canadian C-spine rule for radiography in alert and stable trauma patients. *JAMA*. 2001;286(15):1841–1848.
2. Stiell IG, Clement CM, McKnight RD, et al. The Canadian C-spine rule versus the NEXUS low-risk criteria in patients with trauma. *N Engl J Med*. 2003;349(26):2510–2518.
3. Stiell IG, Clement CM, O'Connor A, et al. Multicentre prospective validation of use of the Canadian C-Spine Rule by triage nurses in the emergency department. *CMAJ*. 2010;182(11):1173–1179.
4. Vaillancourt C, Stiell IG, Beaudoin T, et al. The out-of-hospital validation of the Canadian C-Spine Rule by paramedics. *Ann Emerg Med*. 2009;54(5):663–671.e1.
5. Stiell IG, Clement CM, Grimshaw J, et al. Implementation of the Canadian C-Spine Rule: prospective 12 centre cluster randomized trial. *BMJ*. 2009;339: b4146. doi:10.1136/bmj.b4146.
6. Daffner RH, Hackney DB. ACR Appropriateness Criteria on suspected spine trauma. *J Am Coll Radiol*. 2007;4(11):762–775.

7. Bailitz J, Starr F, Beecroft M, et al. CT should replace three-view radiographs as the initial screening test in patients at high, moderate, and low risk for blunt cervical spine injury: a prospective comparison. *J Trauma*. 2009;66(6):1605–1609.

8. Schenarts PJ, Diaz J, Kaiser C, Carrillo Y, Eddy V, Morris JA Jr. Prospective comparison of admission computed tomographic scan and plain films of the upper cervical spine in trauma patients with altered mental status. *J Trauma*. 2001;51(4):663–668.

12

Magnetic Resonance Imaging for Low Back Pain

MICHAEL E. HOCHMAN

> Although . . . patients preferred [rapid MRI scans to plain radiographs for the evaluation of low back pain], substituting rapid MRI for radiographic evaluations . . . may offer little additional benefit to patients, and it may increase the costs of care because of the increased number of spine operations that patients are likely to undergo.
>
> —JARVIK ET AL.[1]

Research Question: Should patients with low back pain requiring imaging be offered plain radiographs or magnetic resonance imaging (MRI)?[1]

Funding: The Agency for Healthcare Research and Quality and the National Institute for Arthritis and Musculoskeletal and Skin Diseases.

Year Study Began: 1998

Year Study Published: 2003

Study Location: Four imaging sites in Washington State (an outpatient clinic, a teaching hospital, a multispecialty clinic, and a private imaging center)

Who Was Studied: Adults ≥18 years referred by their physician for radio-graphs of the lumbar spine to evaluate lower back pain and/or radiculopathy.

Who Was Excluded: Patients with lumbar surgery within the previous year, those with acute external trauma, and those with metallic implants in the spine.

How Many Patients: 380

Study Overview: See Figure 12.1 for a summary of the trial's design.

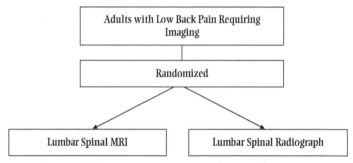

Figure 12.1 Summary of the Trial's Design.

Study Intervention: Patients assigned to the plain radiograph group received the films according to standard protocol. Most patients received anteroposterior and lateral views only, but a small number received additional views when requested by the ordering physician.

Patients assigned to the MRI group were scheduled for the scan on the day of study enrollment whenever possible, and if not, within a week of enrollment. Most scans were performed with a field strength of 1.5 tesla, and all patients received sagittal and axial T2-weighted images (see Figure 12.2).

Follow-Up: 12 months.

Endpoints: Primary outcome: Scores on the 23-item modified Roland-Morris Low Back Pain and Disability Questionnaire (RMLBPDQ).[2] Secondary outcomes: quality of life as assessed using the Medical Outcomes Study 36-Item Short Form Survey (SF-36)[3]; patient satisfaction with care as assessed using the Deyo-Diehl patient satisfaction questionnaire[4]; days of lost work; patient reassurance; and health care resource utilization.

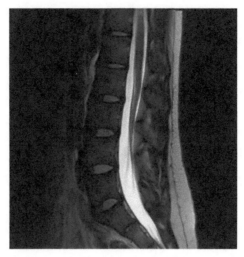

Figure 12.2 Normal sagittal T2 MRI of the lumbar spine.

The 23-item modified RMLBPDQ consists of 23 "yes" or "no" questions. Patients are given 1 point for each "yes" answer for a total possible score of 23. Below are sample questions on the scale:

- I stay at home most of the time because of my back problem or leg pain (sciatica)
- I walk more slowly than usual because of my back problem or leg pain (sciatica)
- I stay in bed most of the time because of my back or leg pain (sciatica)

RESULTS

- The mean age of study patients was 53; 15% were either unemployed, disabled, or on leave from work; 24% had depression; and 70% reported pain radiating to the legs.
- 49% of patients were referred for imaging by primary care doctors, while 51% were referred by specialists.
- The spinal MRI revealed disc herniation in 33% of patients, nerve root impingement in 7%, moderate or severe central canal stenosis in 20%, and lateral recess stenosis in 17%—findings that are typically not detectable with plain radiographs.
- There were no significant differences in back pain scores between the radiograph and MRI groups, though patients in the MRI group were more likely to be reassured by their imaging results; there were no significant differences in total health care costs between the groups (see Tables 12.1 and 12.2).

Table 12.1. THE TRIAL'S KEY FINDINGS AFTER 12 MONTHS[a]

Measure and Outcome	Radiograph Group	MRI Group	P Value
RMLBPDQ (Scale: 0–23)[b]	8.75	9.34	0.53
SF-36, Physical Functioning (Scale: 0–100)[c]	63.77	61.04	not significant[d]
Patient Satisfaction (Scale: 0–11)[c]	7.34	7.04	not significant[d]
Days of Lost Work in Past 4 Weeks	1.26	1.57	not significant[d]
Were you reassured by the imaging results?	58%	74%	0.002

[a] The 12-month outcomes were adjusted for baseline scores; for example, the 12-month Roland scores were adjusted for the fact that, at baseline, scores were slightly higher in patients randomized to the MRI group.
[b] Roland-Morris Low Back Pain and Disability Questionnaire. Higher scores indicate a worse outcome.
[c] Medical Outcomes Study 36-Item Short Form Survey. Higher scores indicate a better outcome.
[d] Actual P value not reported.

Table 12.2. COMPARISON OF RESOURCE UTILIZATION DURING THE STUDY PERIOD

Outcome	Radiograph Group	MRI Group	P Value
Patients Receiving Opioid Analgesics	25%	26%	0.94
Subsequent MRIs per Patient	0.22	0.09	0.01
Physical Therapy, Acupuncture, and Massage Visits per Patient	7.9	3.8	0.008
Specialist Consultations per Patient	0.49	0.73	0.07
Patients Receiving Lumbar Spine Surgery	2%	6%	0.09
Total Costs of Health Care Services	$1,651	$2,121	0.11

Criticisms and Limitations: The increased rate of spinal surgeries and the higher cost of health care services in the MRI group did not reach statistical significance. Therefore, it is not appropriate to draw firm conclusions from these findings.

Other Relevant Studies and Information:

- Other trials have suggested that early spinal imaging (radiographs, computed tomography, and MRI) does not improve outcomes in patients with acute lower back pain without alarm symptoms such as worsening neurologic function,[5] nor does it substantially assist with decision making in patients referred for epidural steroid injections of the spine.[6]

- Guidelines[7] recommend that MRIs of the lumbar spine only be obtained in patients with signs or symptoms of:
  - emergent conditions such as the cauda equina syndrome, tumors, infections, or fractures with neurologic impingement
  - radicular symptoms severe enough and long-lasting enough to warrant surgical intervention
  - spinal stenosis severe enough and long-lasting enough to warrant surgical intervention.

Summary and Implications: Although spinal MRIs (compared with plain radiographs) are reassuring for patients with low back pain, they do not lead to improved functional outcomes. In addition, spinal MRIs detect anatomical abnormalities that would otherwise go undiscovered, possibly leading to spinal surgeries of uncertain value.

CLINICAL CASE: MRI FOR LOW BACK PAIN

Case History:

A 52-year-old man with 6 weeks of low back pain visits your office requesting an MRI of his spine. His symptoms began after doing yard work and have improved only slightly during this time period. The pain is bothersome, but not incapacitating, and radiates down his right leg. He has no systemic symptoms (fevers, chills, or weight loss) and denies bowel or bladder dysfunction. He reports difficulty walking due to the pain. On exam, he is an overweight man in no apparent distress. His range of motion is limited due to pain. He has no neurological deficits.

Based on the results of this trial, should you order an MRI for this patient?

Suggested Answer:

Based on the results of this trial, ordering a spinal MRI in a patient like the one in this vignette is unlikely to lead to improved functional outcomes and may increase the likelihood of spinal surgery by detecting anatomical abnormalities that would otherwise go undiscovered. Still, this trial showed that an MRI may provide reassurance to patients. For this reason, you should reassure your patient in other ways, for example by telling him that he does not have any signs or symptoms of a serious back problem like an infection or cancer.

Other types of spinal imaging such as plain radiographs do not appear to improve outcomes in patients with acute low back pain without alarm symptoms either. Thus, even a plain film may not be necessary at this time.

References

1. Jarvik JG et al. Rapid magnetic resonance imaging vs radiographs for patients with low back pain: a randomized controlled trial. *JAMA*. 2003;289(21):2810–2818.
2. Roland M, Morris R. A study of the natural history of back pain, 1: development of a reliable and sensitive measure of disability in low back pain. *Spine*. 1983;8:141–144.
3. Ware JE, Sherbourne CD. The MOS 36-item short-form survey (SF-36), I: conceptual framework and item selection. *Med Care*. 1992;30:473–483.
4. Deyo RA, Diehl AK. Patient satisfaction with medical care for low-back pain. *Spine*. 1986;11:28–30.
5. Chou R et al. Imaging strategies for low-back pain: systematic review and meta-analysis. *Lancet*. 2009;373(9662):463.
6. Cohen SP et al. Effect of MRI on treatment results or decision making in patients with lumbosacral radiculopathy referred for epidural steroid injections: a multicenter, randomized controlled trial. *Arch Intern Med*. 2012;172(2):134.
7. Bigos SJ et al. *Acute low back pain problems in adults*. Clinical practice guideline No 14. Rockville, MD: Agency for Health Care Policy and Research, Public Health Service, US Department of Health and Human Services, December 1994.

13

Abnormal MRI of the Lumbar Spine without Back Pain

CHRISTOPH I. LEE

> Given the high prevalence of these findings and of back pain, the discovery by MRI of bulges or protrusions in people with low back pain may frequently be coincidental.
>
> —JENSEN ET AL.[1]

Research Question: How prevalent are abnormal findings on MRI scans of the lumbar spine in people without back pain?

Funding: Hoag Memorial Hospital and the Harbor Radiology Research and Education Fund.

Year Study Began: Not reported.

Year Study Published: 1994

Study Location: Single community hospital.

Who Was Studied: Healthy volunteer patients without symptoms of back pain, aged 20–80 years (mean age = 42 years).

Who Was Excluded: Patients with a history of back pain lasting >48 hours or any lumbrosacral radiculopathy.

How Many Patients: 125 (98 asymptomatic, 27 symptomatic)

Study Overview: Prospective cohort study.

Study Intervention: Abnormal MRI scans from 27 people with back pain were selected and mixed randomly with MRI scans from 98 people without back pain. Two neuroradiologists interpreted the scans independently, blinded to clinical information.

Follow-Up: None.

Endpoints: Intervertebral disk findings were classified into the following intervertebral disk categories: normal, bulge (circumferential symmetric extension of the disk beyond the interspace), protrusion (focal of symmetric extension of the disk beyond the interspace), and extrusion (more extreme extension of the disk beyond the interspace). Findings were correlated with level of physical activity (0–4 scale, with 0 indicating no exercise and 4 indicating regular workouts).

RESULTS

- Among the 98 asymptomatic patients, 64% had an intervertebral disk abnormality and 38% had an abnormality at more than one level (Table 13.1).
- Among asymptomatic patients, 52% had at least one intervertebral disk bulge and 27% had at least one disk protrusion (Figure 13.1).
- The prevalence of disk bulges increased with patient age ($P < 0.001$), but the prevalence of disk protrusions did not. The prevalence of disk bulges or protrusions did not vary based on physical activity score.
- The prevalence of disk extrusions in patients with symptomatic back pain was higher than in patients without back pain.

Table 13.1. THE TRIAL'S KEY FINDINGS

Evaluator and Subjects	Bulge n (%)	Protrusion n (%)	Extrusion n (%)
Evaluator 1			
Asymptomatic subjects	52 (53)	30 (31)	2 (2)
Symptomatic subjects	23 (85)	14 (52)	8 (30)
Evaluator 2			
Asymptomatic subjects	50 (51)	23 (23)	0 (0)
Symptomatic subjects	18 (67)	15 (56)	6 (22)
Average of two evaluators			
Asymptomatic subjects	51 (52)	26.5 (27)	1 (1)
Symptomatic subjects	20.5 (76)	14.5 (54)	7 (26)

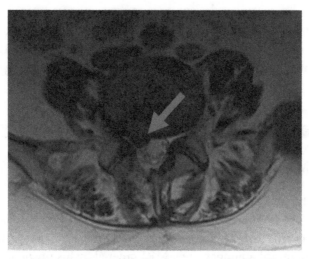

Figure 13.1 Axial T2 MRI image of the lumbar spine with a focal large right L4-L5 disc extrusion within the right lateral recess.

Criticisms and Limitations: Given the small sample size, statistical comparison of people with and without symptoms with regard to the prevalence of disk extrusion was not possible. This study focused on intervertebral disk abnormalities and not other abnormalities that may be the cause of lower back pain, such as facet arthropathy.

Other Relevant Studies and Information:

- Disk "herniation" is used to describe a wide spectrum of abnormalities ranging from a disk bulge to frank extrusion; thus, this term can be misleading and lead to inappropriate interventions.[2] Classification of protrusions and extrusions are more helpful descriptive characteristics.

- The combined task forces of the North American Spine Society, American Society of Spine Radiology, and American Society of Neuroradiology recently published revised and updated guidelines to aid in providing standardized nomenclature and classification of lumbar-disk pathology.[3]
- One study that aimed to determine the value of lumbar spine MRI finding to predict low back pain in asymptomatic subjects found that imaging findings were not predictive of the development or duration of low back pain at 7 years of follow-up.[4]

Summary and Implications: This single cohort study found that many people without back pain have disk bulges or protrusions on MR imaging of the lumbar spine. Given the high prevalence of back pain, these MRI findings are frequently coincidental and their identification and reporting should not directly lead to further diagnostic tests or interventions.

CLINICAL CASE: DISK PROTRUSION ON MRI OF THE LUMBAR SPINE

Case History:

A 42-year-old male presents to your orthopedic clinic to discuss findings from a recent MRI of the lumbar spine. The patient had 3 weeks of low back pain and obtained a lumbar spine MRI ordered by his previous physician. The radiologist reports a 3 mm central disk protrusion at the L3-L4 level and a disk bulge at L4-L5 with mild facet arthropathy. He would like your opinion on whether or not surgery would be helpful.

Suggested Answer:

Jensen et al.[1] found that the discovery of disk bulges and protrusions on lumbar spine MRI are common findings that may be coincidental. A thorough history and physical examination should be obtained to determine whether the patient has any radiculopathy or pain at the reported levels. If the pain cannot be localized to these disk levels, then the findings on MRI are highly likely incidental findings unrelated to the patient's pain. Regardless, without neurological signs and symptoms, conservative therapy should be the first-line treatment plan.

References

1. Jensen MC, Brant-Zawadski MN, Obuchowski N, Modic MT, Malkasian D, Ross JS. Magnetic resonance imaging of the lumbar spine in people without back pain. *N Engl J Med.* 1994;331(2):69–73.
2. Cakir B, Schmidt R, Reichel H, Kafer W. Lumbar disk herniation: what are reliable criterions indicative for surgery? *Orthopedics.* 2009;32(8):589. doi:10.3928/01477447-20090624-19.
3. Fardon DF, Williams AL, Dohring EJ, Murtagh FR, Gabriel Rothman SL, Sze GL. Lumbar disc nomenclature: version 2.0: Recommendations of the combined task forces of the North American Spine Society, the American Society of Spine Radiology and the American Society of Neuroradiology. *Spine J.* 2014;14(11):2525–2545.
4. Borenstein DG, O'Mara JWJr, Boden SD, et al. The value of magnetic resonance imaging of the lumbar spine to predict low-back pain in asymptomatic subjects: a seven-year follow-up study. *J Bone Joint Surg Am.* 2001;83–A(9):1306–1311.

14

Follow-Up MRI for Sciatica

Radiology Outcomes from the Sciatica Trial

CHRISTOPH I. LEE

> . . . in patients who had undergone repeated MRI 1 year after treatment for symptomatic lumbar-disk herniation, anatomical abnormalities that were visible on MRI did not distinguish patients with persistent or recurrent symptoms of sciatica from asymptomatic patients.
>
> —EL BARZOUHI ET AL.[1]

Research Question: Does follow-up MR imaging after 1 year of treatment for a first episode of acute sciatica due to lumbar disk herniation help distinguish between patients with favorable versus unfavorable outcomes?

Funding: The Netherlands Organization for Health Research and Development and the Hoelen Foundation.

Year Study Began: 2002

Year Study Published: 2013

Study Location: Nine medical centers in the Netherlands.

Who Was Studied: Patients 18–65 years of age with a history of 6–12 weeks of sciatica and disk herniation on MRI. Inclusion criteria included a dermatomal

pattern of pain distribution with concurrent neurologic disturbances that cor-
relate with a related nerve root on MRI.

Who Was Excluded: Patients with cauda equina syndrome, muscle paralysis,
or insufficient strength to move against gravity; similar episode of symptoms
during previous 12 months; previous spine surgery; bony stenosis; spondylolis-
thesis; pregnancy; severe comorbidity.

How Many Patients: 283

Study Overview: Multicenter prospective randomized controlled trial. An
early surgery strategy (within 2 weeks after randomization) was compared to
a prolonged conservative care strategy (6 months of conservative therapy followed by surgery if no symptom improvement or request of surgery due to ag-
gravated symptoms). All patients underwent MRI at baseline and after 1 year,
with two experienced neuroradiologists and a neurosurgeon independently
evaluating MRIs while blinded to clinical information.

Study Intervention: Readers decided which disk level showed the most severe
nerve-root compression on MRI, and categorized the disk contour into one of
three categories: disk herniation, bulging disk, and normal disk. The readers
then used a 4-point scale to evaluate the scans for presence of disk herniation
and root compression: 1 for definitely present, 2 for probably present, 3 for possibly present, and 4 for definitely absent.

Follow-Up: Follow-up MRI (1.5 tesla, with and without contrast) 1 year after
enrollment.

Endpoints: Favorable clinical outcome was complete or near complete resolution of symptoms at 1 year on the patient-reported 7-point Likert scale for
global perceived recovery (higher score indicating better recovery). Area under
the receiver-operating characteristic curve was used to assess prognostic accuracy of the 4-point score.

RESULTS

- In the intention-to-treat analysis, a herniated disk was present in 22%
  of patients in the surgery group and 47% of patient in the conservative
  care group at 1-year follow-up ($P < 0.001$) (Table 14.1).
- Readers' ratings assessing the presence of disk herniation on MRI
  (4-point scale) did not distinguish between patients with a favorable

outcome and those with an unfavorable outcome (area under the curve [AUC], 0.48; 95% CI, 0.39–0.58); sensitivity ranged from 0.14–0.32 and specificity ranged from 0.65–0.85.

- At 1-year follow-up, there was no significant difference between the proportion of patients with disk herniation reporting a favorable outcome and proportion of patients with no disk herniation reporting a favorable outcome (85% vs. 83%, respectively; $P = 0.70$).

- After adjusting for randomized treatment, there was no significant association between a favorable outcome at 1 year and MRI-assessed disk herniation, MRI-assessed nerve-root compression, form of disk herniation (protrusion versus extrusion), or size of disk herniation.

Table 14.1. THE TRIAL'S KEY FINDINGS

MRI Finding	Outcome Favorable (n = 224) No. (%)	Unfavorable (n = 43) No. (%)	P Value[a]
Disk herniation			
Present at 1 year	79 (35)	14 (33)	0.70
Size change at 1 year			
Disappeared	143 (64)	28 (65)	0.84
Reduced	66 (29)	9 (21)	0.31
Unchanged	7 (3)	3 (7)	0.23
Enlarged	3 (1)	2 (5)	0.43
No herniation at baseline	5 (2)	1 (2)	0.98
Nerve-root compression			
Present at 1 year	54 (24)	11 (26)	0.87
Visibility on MRI at 1 year			
Disappeared	169 (75)	29 (67)	0.30
Reduced	39 (17)	6 (14)	0.69
Unchanged	13 (6)	6 (14)	0.06
Increased	3 (1)	2 (5)	0.43

[a] P value for difference in proportions between favorable outcome and unfavorable outcome groups (significant at $P < 0.05$).

Criticisms and Limitations: There was only moderate agreement among the three readers for MRI assessment of disk herniation (k = 0.57–0.67) and nerve-root compression (k = 0.46–0.74). Clinical and imaging outcomes were only determined at the 1-year mark after randomization and no other time points.

Other Relevant Studies and Information:

- The most common cause of sciatica is a herniated disk and most cases resolve spontaneously with conservative treatment. Patients who fail conservative treatment may be offered surgery; however, randomized controlled trials have shown that 15%–20% of surgery patients report recurring or persistent symptoms.[2,3]
- Imaging findings of disk herniation are known to persist for years on MRI even after disk surgery and resolution of symptoms.[4]
- This group's previous report of clinical outcomes from the randomized controlled trial showed that early surgery led to faster recovery when compared with conservative therapy, but there were no significant differences in clinical outcomes at 1 year between the two groups.[3]
- A recent meta-analysis suggests that there is no conclusive evidence for the diagnostic accuracy of MRI for acute sciatica.[5]

Summary and Implications: The presence of disk herniation on MRI at 1-year follow-up after treatment for sciatica does not help distinguish between favorable and unfavorable clinical outcomes (Figure 14.1). Thus, follow-up imaging

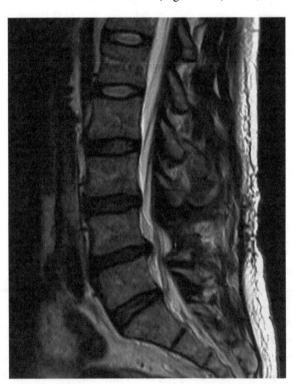

Figure 14.1 Sagittal T2 fat saturation MRI image of the lumbar spine with recurrent posterior L4-L5 disc protrusion 1 year status post discectomy at this location.

(after the first episode of acute sciatica) for patients with persistent or recurrent sciatica symptoms after treatment may not lead to helpful diagnostic information.

CLINICAL CASE: SCIATICA IMAGING

Case History:

A 56-year-old male patient with a history of sciatica status post unilateral discectomy returns to your office complaining of persistent radiating pain down his left leg. The patient is 10 months removed from his surgery and has minimal relief. He requests a follow-up MRI to determine if his lumbar disk herniation has returned. He reports no new symptoms and his neurological examination is intact. How should you counsel the patient about further imaging?

Suggested Answer:

Based on the radiology outcomes of the Sciatica Trial, it is unlikely that follow-up MRI 1 year after treatment will aid in management decisions. Any abnormalities seen may be coincidental and result in additional surgical treatment or other procedures that are unnecessary.[6] You should advise your patient that there is no evidence that suggests that repeat imaging would be helpful in his scenario, and that treatment options would remain the same with or without follow-up imaging.

References

1. el Barzouhi A, Vleggeert-Lankamp CL, Lycklama à Nijeholt GJ, et al. Magnetic resonance imaging in follow-up assessment of sciatica. *N Engl J Med*. 2013;368(11):999–1007.
2. Arts MP, Brand R, van den Akker ME, Koes BW, Bartels RH, Peul WC; Leiden-The Hague Spine Intervention Prognostic Study Group (SIPS). Tubular diskectomy vs conventional microdiskectomy for sciatica: a randomized controlled trial. *JAMA*. 2009;302(2):149–158.
3. Peul WC, van Houwelingen HC, van den Hout WB, et al. Surgery versus prolonged conservative treatment for sciatica. *N Engl J Med*. 2007;356(22):2245–2256.
4. Barth M, Diepers M, Weiss C, Thomé C. Two-year outcome after lumbar microdiscectomy versus microscopic sequestrectomy: part 2: radiographic evaluation and correlation with clinical outcome. *Spine (Phila Pa 1976)*. 2008;33(3):273–279.
5. Wassenaar M, van Rijn RM, van Tulder MW, et al. Magnetic resonance imaging for diagnosing lumbar spinal pathology in adult patients with low back pain or sciatica: a diagnostic systematic review. *Eur Spine J*. 2012;21(2):220–227.
6. Lurie JD, Birkmeyer NJ, Weinstein JN. Rates of advanced spinal imaging and spine surgery. *Spine (Phila Pa 1976)*. 2003;28(6):616–620.

15

Early Imaging for Back Pain in Older Adults

Back Pain Outcomes Using Longitudinal Data (BOLD) Study

CHRISTOPH I. LEE

> Among older adults with a new primary care visit for back pain, early imaging was not associated with better 1-year outcomes.
>
> —JARVIK ET AL.[1]

Research Question: Is there benefit for early imaging of older adults presenting with new onset back pain without radiculopathy?

Funding: Agency for Healthcare Research and Quality and the NIH Intramural Research Program.

Year Study Began: 2011

Year Study Published: 2015

Study Location: Primary or urgent care centers from three integrated US health care systems: Harvard Vanguard, Henry Ford Health System, and Kaiser Permanente Northern California.

Who Was Studied: Adults ≥65 years with a new primary care visit for low back pain, defined as no prior visit for low back pain within the previous 6 months.

Who Was Excluded: Patients with a health care encounter for back pain within the previous 6 months; prior lumbar spine surgery; developmental spine deformity; inflammatory spondyloarthropathy; spinal malignancy or infection; history of cancer within past 5 years except non-melanomatous skin cancer; history of HIV within past 5 years; no telephone; planning to leave health care system within 12 months; non-English speaking; severe mental impairment.

How Many Patients: 5,239

Study Overview: Prospective observational cohort study. Patients who obtained early imaging (lumbar spine imaging within 6 weeks of their index visit) were matched 1:1 with controls who did not obtain early imaging using propensity score matching of demographic and clinical characteristics, including diagnosis, pain severity, functional status, and prior resource use.

Exposure: The main exposure was diagnostic imaging (x-rays, CT, and MRI) of the thoracic or lumbar spine within six weeks of the index visit. Early imaging patients were separated into two cohorts: patient undergoing early plain film imaging, and patients undergoing early advanced imaging (CT or MRI).

Follow-Up: 3-, 6-, and 12-month follow-up after study enrollment.

Endpoints: The primary outcome measured was 12-month back or leg pain–related disability measured by the modified Roland-Morris Disability Questionnaire (RMDQ; score range 0–24, with 0 indicating no pain-related limitations and 24 indicating maximal pain-related disability). Additional secondary endpoints included ratings of average back pain intensity in the past week, average leg pain intensity in the past week, back pain interference with general activity, depression and anxiety, health status measures, and a measure for injury due to falls.

RESULTS

- There were no clinically or statistically significant differences in the primary outcome measures (RMDQ score) between early and not early imaging groups (x-ray and CT/MRI) at any time point.
- There were no clinically meaningful differences in secondary patient-reported outcomes (e.g., pain intensity, health status measures) between the early imaging (x-ray and CT/MRI) and control groups at 12 months.

- Mean total resource utilization (in relative value units) was 40% higher ($P < 0.001$) in the early radiograph and 50% higher ($P = 0.01$) in the early CT/MRI group that in the no early imaging groups; overall costs were 27% ($P < 0.001$) and 30% ($P < 0.04$) higher, respectively (Table 15.1).
- There was no significant difference in the incidence of missed cancer diagnoses with or without early imaging on 1-year follow-up; only 1 cancer was detected by early imaging and this was not located in the spine but in adjacent adenopathy.

Table 15.1. THE TRIAL'S KEY FINDINGS

Imaging Group and Follow-Up Period	RMDQ[a] Matched Control Mean (SD)	RMDQ Early Imaging Mean (SD)	P Value[b]
Radiograph			
n	1,174	1,174	
3 months	9.54 (6.64)	9.54 (6.41)	0.93
6 months	9.06 (6.88)	8.92 (6.57)	0.66
12 months	8.74 (6.95)	8.54 (6.56)	0.36
CT/MRI			
n	349	349	0.76
3 months	11.50 (6.82)	11.60 (6.51)	0.15
6 months	11.20 (7.13)	10.50 (6.66)	0.18
12 months	10.50 (7.20)	9.81 (6.99)	

[a] RMDQ = Roland-Morris Disability Questionnaire.
[b] *P* value from linear mixed-effects models to obtain adjusted differences between those who received early imaging and those who did not, adjusting for age, sex, diagnosis, back pain duration, and total relative value units (RVUs) in the year prior to index visit.

Criticisms and Limitations: Even with propensity matching, there was potential for confounding by indication (e.g., worse prognoses in the early imaging group versus no early imaging group). Patterns of care may have varied by site, confounding utilization measures. Baseline measures were obtained up to 3 weeks after the index visit, and responses could reflect response to therapy since that visit.

Other Relevant Studies and Information:

- Approximately 90% of older adults have incidental findings on spine imaging, which may lead to inappropriate interventions and associated increased morbidity (Figure 15.1).[2]

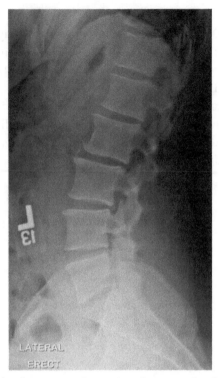

Figure 15.1 Lateral lumbar spine radiograph with scattered mild degenerative changes throughout the lumbar spine. No definite etiology is seen on this radiograph to explain the patient's chronic lower back pain symptoms.

- As of May 2015, the ACR Appropriateness Criteria still considers early imaging with MRI of the lumbar spine without contrast to be appropriate for patients >70 years of age who have no other "red flag" conditions (e.g., cancer, infection, cauda equina syndrome).[3]
- The American College of Physicians recommends against diagnostic imaging for patients with low back pain in the absence of severe progressive neurologic deficits or signs or symptoms that suggest a serious or specific underlying condition.[4]

Summary and Implications: Early imaging for new onset back pain among older adults presenting to primary care was not associated with improved patient-reported outcomes at 1-year follow-up. However, patients undergoing early imaging had substantially higher resource use and reimbursement expenditures than did patients not undergoing early imaging for new onset back pain.

CLINICAL CASE: BACK PAIN IN OLDER ADULT

Case History:
A 74-year-old female patient presents to your primary care clinic with new onset low back pain, 4 weeks in duration. She does not recall an acute injury or other trigger, and has been self-medicating with nonsteroidal anti-inflammatory drugs. She is otherwise in good health, and is being treated for mild hypertension and hyperlipidemia. Her vital signs are normal and her neurological exam is intact. What further diagnostic tests, if any, are indicated?

Suggested Answer:
This study suggests that early imaging should not be performed routinely for new onset back pain regardless of age. Even though some guidelines consider imaging for acute back pain in the elderly to be appropriate, more evidence points to no benefit in 1-year patient-reported outcomes with the potential for harm from interventions for incidental imaging findings. No diagnostic imaging should be pursued, and conservative management with analgesics and potentially physical therapy should be pursued.

References

1. Jarvik JG, Gold LS, Comstock BA, et al. Association of early imaging for back pain with clinical outcomes in older adults. *JAMA*. 2015;313(11):1143–1153.
2. Jarvik JJ, Hollingworth W, Heagerty P, Haynor DR, Deyo RA. The Longitudinal Assessment of Imaging and Disability of the Back (LAIDBack) Study. *Spine (Phila Pa 1976)*. 2001;26(10):1158–1166.
3. Chou R, Qaseem A, Owens DK, Shekelle P; Clinical Guidelines Committee of the American College of Physicians. Diagnostic imaging for low back pain: advice for high-value health care from the American College of Physicians. *Ann Intern Med*. 2011;154(3):181–189.
4. American College of Radiology. ACR appropriateness criteria for low back pain. http://www.acr.org/~/media/ACR/Documents/AppCriteria/Diagnostic/LowBackPain.pdf. Published 1996. Updated 2015. Accessed May 1, 2015.

SECTION 3

Chest Pain

16

Computed Tomography for Pulmonary Embolism

The Prospective Investigation of Pulmonary Embolism Diagnosis (PIOPED) II Trial

CHRISTOPH I. LEE

> The predictive value of either CTA or CTA-CTV is high with a concordant clinical assessment, but additional testing is necessary when clinical probability is inconsistent with the imaging results.
>
> —STEIN ET AL.[1]

Research Question: How accurate is multidetector computed tomographic angiography (CTA) with or without venous phase imaging (CTV) for diagnosing acute pulmonary embolism (PE)?

Funding: National Heart, Lung, and Blood Institute.

Year Study Began: 2001

Year Study Published: 2006

Study Location: Eight North American (US and Canada) tertiary medical centers.

Who Was Studied: Patients ≥18 years of age and clinically suspected acute PE referred for diagnostic imaging for suspected PE or had consultation requests for suspected PE.

Who Was Excluded: Patients who were unable to complete testing within 36 hours, abnormal creatinine levels, long-term renal dialysis, critically ill, on ventilator support, allergic to contrast agents, myocardial infarction within preceding month, possible or confirmed pregnancy, inferior vena cava (IVC) filter in situ, no suspected PE, upper extremity DVT, previously enrolled in the study, ventricular fibrillation or sustained ventricular tachycardia within 24 hours, shock or hypotension, planned thrombolytic therapy within next 24 hours, < 8 years of age, incarcerated.

How Many Patients: 824

Study Overview: All patients underwent clinical assessment of the probability of PE (Wells score) (Table 16.1).[2] All patients consented to diagnostic imaging evaluations (as detailed in the Diagnostic Evaluation section). A composite reference standard was used to confirm diagnosis of PE.

Diagnostic Evaluation: All patients consented to multidetector CTA-CTV, ventilation/perfusion (V/Q) scanning, venous compression ultrasonography of lower extremities, and, if necessary, pulmonary digital subtraction angiography (DSA). Pulmonary DSA was reserved for patients in whom PE was not conclusively diagnosed or ruled out with noninvasive tests.

Table 16.1. Wells Score for Clinical Probability of PE

Clinical Feature	Score[a]
DVT signs and symptoms (leg swelling, pain with palpation)	3.0
Heart rate >100 beats/minute	1.5
Immobilized ≥3 consecutive days or surgery in previous 4 weeks	1.5
Previous objectively diagnosed PE or DVT	1.5
Hemoptysis	1.0
Cancer (with treatment within past 6 months or palliative treatment)	1.0
PE more likely than alternative diagnoses on basis of history, physical examination, ECG, blood tests, and chest x-ray	3.0

[a] Total score <2.0 indicates low probability, 2.0–6.0 indicates moderate probability, >6.0 indicates high probability. PE = pulmonary embolism; DVT = deep venous thrombosis; ECG = electrocardiography.

Follow-Up: Telephone interviews with patients 3 and 6 months after enrollment for patients in whom PE was ruled out by the reference test.

Endpoints: Sensitivity, specificity, and positive predictive value (PPV) of CTA alone and CTA-CTV for diagnosing acute PE were calculated. Diagnosis of PE according to the reference standard required one of the following (with two-reader agreement): V-Q scan shows high probability of PE in patient with no history of PE, abnormal pulmonary DSA, abnormal venous ultrasound in patient without previous DVT and nondiagnostic V-Q scan. Exclusion of PE according to the reference standard required one of the following: normal pulmonary DSA, normal V-Q scan, low or very low probability V-Q scan in combination with clinical Wells score <2 and normal venous ultrasound.

RESULTS

- Of the 824 patients who received a reference diagnosis, 192 (23%) were diagnosed with acute PE.
- Two of the 590 patients (<1%) with interpretable CTA initially ruled out for PE who did not receive anticoagulation had clinical courses consistent with unrecognized PE after 6 months of follow-up.
- Poor imaging quality led to inconclusive results for 6.2% (51/824) of CTA studies and 10.6% (87/824) of CTA-CTV studies.
- Excluding studies with poor imaging quality, CTA had 83% sensitivity (95% CI, 76%–92%) and 96% specificity (95% CI, 93%–97%) for diagnosing acute PE, and CTA-CTV had 90% sensitivity (95% CI, 84%–93%) and 95% specificity (95% CI, 92%–96%) (Table 16.2).
- CTA had a PPV of 96% with concordantly high probability on clinical assessment, and 92% with intermediate probability on clinical assessment.

Table 16.2. THE TRIAL'S KEY FINDINGS[a]

Predictive Value	Clinical Probability (%)		
	High Value (95% CI)	Intermediate Value (95% CI)	LowValue (95% CI)
PPV of CTA	96 (78–99)	92 (84–96)	58 (40–73)
PPV of CTA or CTV	96 (81–99)	90 (82–94)	57 (40–72)
NPV of CTA	60 (32–83)	89 (82–93)	96 (92–98)
NPV of CTA + CTV	82 (48–97)	92 (85–96)	97 (92–98)

[a] PPV= positive predictive value; NPV = negative predictive value; CTA = computed tomography angiography; CTV = computed tomography venography.

Criticisms and Limitations: The composite reference standard used is not an absolute standard for diagnosis of acute PE. If poor imaging quality studies were included, then sensitivity of diagnostic CTA and CTA-CTV would be lower. The reported values may not be applicable to pregnant patients, renal failure patients, or critically ill patients.

Other Relevant Studies and Information:

- Since the majority of patients with PE also have deep venous thrombosis, venous-phase multidetector CTV can be acquired in combination with CTA for improved disease detection.[3–5]
- Normal D-dimer test among patients with a low or intermediate clinical probability of PE can safely be used to eliminate the need for diagnostic imaging if D-dimer is measured with a sensitive test (e.g., rapid ELISA).[6]
- A meta-analysis of the literature suggests that it appears to be safe to withhold anticoagulation after negative CTA results.[7]
- The American College of Emergency Physicians clinical policy guidelines indicate that for patients with a low pretest probability for PE (Wells score ≤ 4) who require additional diagnostic testing (e.g., positive D-dimer result, or highly sensitive D-dimer test not available), a negative multidetector CT pulmonary angiogram alone can be used to exclude PE.[8]
- The American College of Radiology gives high appropriateness scores for the use of CTA (9 out of 9) and ultrasound of the lower extremities with Doppler (7 out of 9) in cases of suspected pulmonary embolism. CTA-CTV is given an intermediate score (6 out of 9) in cases of suspected pulmonary embolism.[9]

Summary and Implications: Combined multidetector CTA-CTV has higher sensitivity for diagnosing acute PE than CTA alone, with similar specificity (Figure 16.1). The positive predictive value of both CTA and CTA-CTV is high with concordant clinical assessments. However, additional testing is indicated when CTA imaging findings and clinical assessment are discordant.

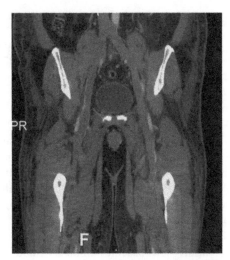

Figure 16.1 Coronal contrast enhanced CT venogram of the pelvis and thighs with extensive deep venous thrombosis extending superiorly from the lower extremities into the iliac veins and the lower IVC to the level of the partially visualized IVC filter. Image courtesy of David S. Wang, MD: Stanford University.

CLINICAL CASE: IMAGING FOR ACUTE PULMONARY EMBOLISM

Case History:

A 48-year-old male presents to the emergency department with acute chest pain after traveling 6 hours on a transcontinental flight. On physical examination, he is tachycardic (pulse = 110) with all other vital signs in the normal range. His ECG and standard laboratory results are unremarkable. His history is notable for a broken ankle repaired 3 weeks ago for which the patient currently has a cast, and a remote history of prior lower extremity DVT. A CTA study of adequate image quality showed no evidence of acute PE. Should PE be ruled out in this patient at this point, or is additional imaging required?

Suggested Answer:

This patient has moderate clinical probability of having an acute PE based on his Wells score (4.5). Given the 17% false-negative rate for CTA and the current level of clinical suspicion, lower extremity imaging is indicated. Based on this study, CTA-CTV has higher sensitivity than CTA alone with equal specificity. Both CTV and ultrasound would be appropriate in this instance, with the latter preferable since the patient just had a contrast injection for the CTA study and CTV could be compromised by artifact from the ankle cast.

References

1. Stein PD, Fowler SE, Goodman LR, et al. Multidetector computed tomography for acute pulmonary embolism. *N Eng J Med*. 2006;354(22):2317–2327.
2. Wells PS, Anderson DR, Rodger M, et al. Excluding pulmonary embolism at the bedside without diagnostic imaging: management of patients with suspected pulmonary embolism presenting to the emergency department by using a simple clinical model and D-dimer. *Ann Intern Med*. 2001;135(2):98–107.
3. Loud PA, Katz DS, Bruce DA, Klippenstein DL, Grossman ZD. Deep venous thrombosis with suspected pulmonary embolism: detection with combined CT venography and pulmonary angiography. *Radiology*. 2001;219(2):498–502.
4. Cham MD, Yankelevitz DF, Henschke CI. Thromboembolic disease detection at indirect CT venography versus CT pulmonary angiography. *Radiology* 2005;234(2): 591–594.
5. Stein PD, Matta F, Yaekoub AY, et al. CT venous phase venography with 64-slice CT angiography in the diagnosis of acute pulmonary embolism. *Clin Appl Thromb Hemost*. 2010;16(4):422–429.
6. Perrier A, Roy P-M, Sanchez O, et al. Multidetector-row computed tomography in suspected pulmonary embolism. *N Engl J Med*. 2005;352(17):1760–1768.
7. Moores LK, Jackson WLJr, Shorr AF, Jackson JL. Meta-analysis: outcomes in patients with suspected pulmonary embolism managed with computed tomographic pulmonary angiography. *Ann Intern Med*. 2004;141(11):866–874.
8. Fesmire FM, Brown MD, Espinosa JA, et al. Critical issues in the evaluation and management of adult patients presenting to the emergency department with suspected pulmonary embolism. *Ann Emerg Med* 2011;57(6):628–652.
9. Bettman MA, Baginski SG, White RD, et al. ACR appropriateness criteria® acute chest pain—suspected pulmonary embolism. *J Thorac Imaging*. 2012;27(2):W28–W31.

17

Diagnosing Acute Pulmonary Embolism

The Christopher Study

MICHAEL E. HOCHMAN

> This large cohort study of . . . patients with clinically suspected pulmonary embolism demonstrates that the use of [simple clinical criteria], D-dimer testing, and CT scan can guide treatment decisions.
> —THE CHRISTOPHER STUDY INVESTIGATORS[1]

Research Question: Can a simple predefined protocol involving clinical criteria (the modified Wells criteria), D-dimer testing, and computed tomography (CT) safely and effectively rule out acute pulmonary embolism (PE) among patients who are clinically suspected of this condition?[1]

Funding: An unrestricted grant from participating hospitals.

Year Study Began: 2002

Year Study Published: 2006

Study Location: 12 centers in the Netherlands.

Who Was Studied: Adults ≥18 years with clinically suspected acute PE. Patients presenting to the emergency room (81.7%) as well as hospitalized patients (18.3%) were included. Patients were required to have "sudden onset of dyspnea, sudden deterioration of existing dyspnea, or sudden onset of pleuritic chest pain without another apparent cause."

Who Was Excluded: Patients receiving treatment doses of unfractionated or low-molecular-weight heparin for >24 hours, those with a life expectancy <3 months, those who were pregnant, those with an allergy to IV contrast, those with renal insufficiency (a creatinine clearance <30 mL/s), or those with hemodynamic instability.

How Many Patients: 3,306

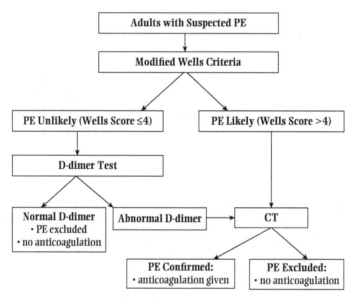

Figure 17.1 Summary of Christopher's Protocol.

Study Overview: See Figure 17.1 for a summary of Christopher's Protocol.

Study Intervention: Patients with a suspected PE were evaluated by an attending physician. Pulmonary embolism was categorized as either "unlikely" if the modified Wells score was ≤4 or "likely" if the score was >4 (Table 17.1).

Table 17.1. MODIFIED WELLS SCORE[a]

Criteria	Points
Signs and symptoms of DVT (e.g., leg swelling and tenderness of deep veins)	3.0
PE more likely than alternative diagnoses	3.0
Heart rate >100 beats per minute	1.5
Immobilization for more than 3 days or surgery in previous 4 weeks	1.5
History of PE or DVT	1.5
Hemoptysis	1.0
Active malignancy within previous 6 months	1.0

[a]Wells PS et al. Derivation of a simple clinical model to categorize patients' probability of pulmonary embolism: increasing the model's utility with the SimpliRED D-dimer. *Thromb Haemost.* 2000;83:416–420.

Patients with a modified Wells score ≤4 underwent D-dimer testing, and if the test was negative (D-dimer concentration ≤500 ng/mL), the diagnosis of PE was considered excluded and anticoagulant treatment was withheld. If the D-dimer test was positive, the patient was referred for a CT angiogram of the chest (see Table 17.2). In addition, patients with a modified Wells score >4 were referred for chest CT.

When a PE was diagnosed with CT, patients received anticoagulation with unfractionated heparin or low-molecular-weight heparin followed by warfarin. When the CT did not demonstrate acute PE, anticoagulation was withheld

Table 17.2. CHRISTOPHER'S KEY FINDINGS

Patient Groups	Nonfatal Thromboembolic Events (95% CI)	Fatal Thromboembolic Events (95% CI)
PE excluded with Wells criteria and D-dimer (32% of patients)	0.5% (0.2%–1.1%)	0% (0.0%–0.3%)
PE excluded with CT (46% of patients)	1.3% (0.7%–2.0%)	0.5% (0.2%–1.0%)
PE confirmed with CT (20% of patients)	3.0% (1.8%–4.6%)[a]	1.6% (0.8%–2.9%)[a]
CT not performed or inconclusive (2% of patients)	2.9%[b]	1.4%[b]

[a] Refers to recurrent symptomatic thromboembolic events.
[b] 95% confidence intervals not reported.

and alternative diagnoses were considered. For inconclusive CT results (i.e., motion artifact or inadequate contrast enhancement), patients were managed according to the discretion of the attending physician.

Follow-Up: 3 months.

Endpoints: Primary outcome: Symptomatic venous thromboembolic events (fatal or nonfatal PE or deep venous thrombosis [DVT]).

RESULTS

Modified Wells Criteria and D-dimer Classifications:

- 66.7% of patients had a modified Wells score ≤4 and underwent D-dimer testing.
- 52% of patients who underwent D-dimer testing had a positive result.
- 68% of all patients were referred for a CT scan either because of an abnormal D-dimer test or because of a modified Wells score >4.

CT Scan Results among Patients Referred for CT:

- 30% of patients were found to have a PE and received anticoagulation.
- 67% of patients were found not to have a PE, and anticoagulation was withheld unless there were other indications for anticoagulation.
- 3% of patients had inconclusive results or did not receive the CT scan; in 10% of these situations the physician elected to start anticoagulation.
- See Table 17.2 for key findings.

Criticisms and Limitations: A high percentage of study patients (68%) ultimately required CT scans for evaluation; that is, the protocol only prevented 32% of patients from receiving a CT.

The study did not compare alternative protocols for evaluating patients with suspected pulmonary emboli; therefore it is not known how this protocol compares with other protocols.

Other Relevant Studies and Information:

- Another study involving a different, more complicated protocol also showed the potential utility of clinical assessment, D-dimer testing, and imaging for assessing patients with suspected pulmonary emboli.[2]

- The PIOPED I study showed that ventilation/perfusion (V/Q) lung scans can be helpful in confirming a PE when there is both a high clinical probability and a high radiologic suspicion for a PE. In addition, V-Q scans are helping in excluding a PE when the scan is normal and when there is a low clinical probability. However, in many cases the clinical and radiologic results after V-Q scanning are contradictory and/or inconclusive.[3]

- The PIOPED II study showed that CT angiography, when combined with a clinical assessment (traditional Wells criteria), accurately confirms or excludes the diagnosis of PE except when the clinical assessment and radiologic results are contradictory.[4]

- The traditional Wells criteria, which use a scoring system similar to the system used in the Christopher study, categorize patients as low, intermediate, or high probability for PE.[5]

Summary and Implications: A simple protocol involving clinical criteria (the modified Wells criteria), D-dimer testing, and CT (see Figure 17.2) can safely and effectively exclude acute PE in patients who are clinically suspected of the condition. Patients who followed the protocol, which is shown in Figure 17.1, had very low rates of subsequent thromboembolic events at 3-month follow-up.

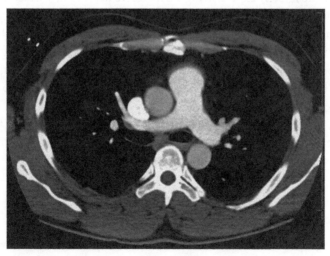

Figure 17.2 Normal contrast-enhanced pulmonary embolus protocol CT of the chest.

CLINICAL CASE: DIAGNOSING ACUTE PULMONARY EMBOLISM

Case History:

An 85-year-old man with congestive heart failure, chronic kidney disease, and a distant history of colon cancer presents to the emergency room with the relatively acute onset of worsening shortness of breath over the past 12 hours. He has had several emergency room visits and hospitalizations for heart failure exacerbations and pneumonia over the past year.

On exam, the patient has a heart rate of 110 and a respiratory rate of 24. He has elevated neck veins and bilateral lower extremity swelling.

Based on the results of the Christopher study, how should you evaluate this patient for a pulmonary embolism?

Suggested Answer:

According to the Christopher study, patients with a suspected diagnosis of pulmonary embolism and a modified Wells score ≤4 should receive D-dimer testing to evaluate for pulmonary embolism. If the D-dimer is elevated, they should receive a chest CT scan to confirm or refute the diagnosis. In contrast, patients with a modified Wells score >4 should immediately receive a chest CT.

The patient in this vignette is complicated: although he presents with the sudden onset of dyspnea, an alternative diagnosis—congestive heart failure—may be a more likely cause of his symptoms. If you believe that this patient is most likely experiencing a congestive heart failure exacerbation, it would probably not be appropriate to evaluate him for a pulmonary embolism at all, because only patients with clinically suspected acute pulmonary embolism were included in the Christopher study. In fact, evaluating him for a pulmonary embolism could be harmful: 68% of patients in the Christopher study ultimately underwent a CT scan, which could be damaging to his kidneys because of the contrast load.

Thus, although the Christopher study provides a helpful protocol for evaluating patients with a suspected pulmonary embolism, clinical judgment remains critical for ensuring that the protocol is used appropriately.

References

1. Christopher Study Investigators. Effectiveness of managing suspected pulmonary embolism using an algorithm combining clinical probability, D-dimer testing, and computed tomography. *JAMA*. 2006;295(2):172–179.

2. Perrier A et al. Multidetector-row computed tomography in suspected pulmonary embolism. *N Engl J Med*. 2005;352(17):1760–1768.
3. The PIOPED Investigators. Value of the ventilation/perfusion scan in acute pulmonary embolism: results of the prospective investigation of pulmonary embolism diagnosis (PIOPED). *JAMA*. 1990;263(20):2753–2759.
4. Stein PD et al. Multidetector computed tomography for acute pulmonary embolism. *N Engl J Med*. 2006;354(22):2317–2327.
5. Wells PS et al. Excluding pulmonary embolism at the bedside without diagnostic imaging: management of patients with suspected pulmonary embolism presenting to the emergency department by using a simple clinical model and D-dimer. *Ann Intern Med*. 2001;135:98–107.

18

CT Angiography versus V/Q Scans to Rule Out Pulmonary Embolism

CHRISTOPH I. LEE

> In this study, CTA was not inferior to V/Q scanning in ruling out pulmonary embolism.
>
> —ANDERSON ET AL.[1]

Research Question: Is CT angiography (CTA) a reliable alterative to ventilation/perfusion (V/Q) scans as an initial noninvasive imaging examination for excluding the diagnosis of acute PE?

Funding: Canadian Institutes of Health Research.

Year Study Began: 2001

Year Study Published: 2007

Study Location: Five tertiary medical centers (4 Canadian, 1 US).

Who Was Studied: Adult patients likely to have acute PE based on a Wells clinical model score of ≥4.5 or a positive D-dimer assay.

Who Was Excluded: DVT or PE diagnosed within previous 3 months; no change in pulmonary symptoms within previous 2 weeks; parenteral anticoagulant use >48 hours; comorbidity with life expectancy <3 months; contraindication to IV contrast (renal insufficiency); long-term use of anticoagulants; pregnant; <18 years of age; geographic inaccessibility to follow-up.

How Many Patients: 1,147

Study Overview: Randomized controlled investigator-blinded noninferiority clinical trial, with V/Q scan representing the standard of care.

Interventions: All patients underwent a clinical pretest probability assignment by a physician using the Wells model, along with a D-dimer assay. Patients who were clinically considered to have a higher likelihood of PE (Wells score ≥ 4.5) or a positive D-dimer assay were then randomized to undergo either V/Q scan or CTA.

Follow-Up: Patients initially excluded for acute PE after imaging were followed for a 3-month period, with clinic or telephone follow-up at 1 week and 3 months after initial presentation.

Endpoints: Primary outcome was development of symptomatic PE or proximal DVT in patients for whom PE was initially excluded.

RESULTS

- Among the evaluable patients, 19.2% (133/694) in the CTA group and 14.2% (101/712) in the V/Q scan group were initially diagnosed with acute PE and treated with anticoagulation (difference, 5.0%; 95% CI, 1.1%–8.9%) (Table 18.1).
- Among patients initially ruled out for having acute PE, 0.4% (2/561) in the CTA group and 1.0% (6/611) in the V/Q scan group developed venous thromboembolism (PE or DVT) at 3-month follow-up (difference, –0.6%, 95% CI, –1.6% to 0.3%), with 1 fatal PE in the V/Q scan group.
- In the V/Q scan group, 54.2% (386/712) had nondiagnostic scan results. Of these, 16 (4.1%) had DVT found on ultrasound and 10 (2.6%) had PE diagnosed by CTA or conventional angiography in the initial baseline diagnostic period.

- Among patients in the CTA group with technically adequate scan results ruling out acute PE, 1.3% (7/531) were found to have DVT on ultrasound in the initial baseline diagnostic period and were treated with anticoagulation.

Table 18.1. THE TRIAL'S KEY FINDINGS

Venous Thromboembolism	CTA (n = 694)	V/Q (n = 712)	Absolute Difference % (95% CI)
Baseline			
PE alone	94 (13.5%)	64 (9.0%)	
PE and DVT	29 (4.2%)	19 (2.7%)	
DVT	10 (1.4%)	18 (2.5%)	
Total	133 (19.2%)	101 (14.2%)	5.0% (1.1%–8.9%)
3-Month Follow-Up			
PE	2 (0.4%)	4 (0.7%)	
DVT	0 (0%)	2 (0.3%)	
Total	2 (0.4%)	6 (1.0%)	−0.6% (−1.6% to 0.34%)

PE = pulmonary embolism; DVT = deep venous thrombosis; CTA = CT pulmonary angiography; V/Q = ventilation-perfusion scan.

Criticisms and Limitations: Clinicians in the study were less comfortable excluding PE in patients with nondiagnostic V/Q scans than with negative CTA examinations, with some crossover between groups. The vast majority (89%) of patients were outpatients; thus results cannot be generalized to inpatient populations. Two different CT protocols were used, with 72% of CTA patients undergoing multidetector CTA and 28% undergoing single-detector CTA.

Other Relevant Studies and Information:

- This study confirms results from prior cohort studies finding a combination of negative CTA and lower extremity ultrasound safely excludes diagnosis of acute PE and that these patients do not require anticoagulation.[2-4]
- V/Q scans still have a role in ruling out acute PE, given the associated lower radiation dose and fewer adverse events and contraindications. A negative V/Q scan effectively rules out acute PE if clinical suspicion is low.[5]

- The American College of Emergency Physicians clinical policy guidelines give a level "B" grade recommendation for the use of a negative multidetector CT pulmonary angiography study in a patient with low clinical probability (Wells score ≤ 4) to effectively rule out acute PE, as well as a level "B" recommendation for venous ultrasound as the initial imaging modality in the emergency department for suspected thromboembolism.[6]
- The American College of Radiology gives high appropriateness scores for the use of CTA (9 out of 9), V/Q scans (8 out of 9), and ultrasound of the lower extremities with Doppler (7 out of 9) in cases of suspected pulmonary embolism.[7]

Summary and Implications: A strategy to rule out PE (and the need for anticoagulation therapy) using clinical probability, D-dimer, and lower extremity ultrasound in conjunction with either CTA or V/Q scanning resulted in low, similar rates of venous thromboembolic events at 3 months of follow-up. However, more patients were diagnosed with acute PE in the CTA arm (Figure 18.1); further research is required to confirm whether some pulmonary emboli detected by CTA are clinically irrelevant.

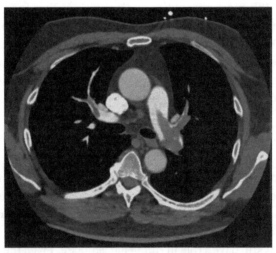

Figure 18.1 Axial contrast enhanced PE protocol CT image with large proximal pulmonary emboli bilaterally.

CLINICAL CASE: CTA VERSUS V/Q TO RULE OUT PE

Case History:
A 36-year-old female presents to the emergency department with acute chest pain and shortness of breath. She has recently had a diagnosis of breast cancer for which she had a modified radical mastectomy within the last month and is undergoing systemic therapy. She has tachycardia on physical examination and mild pain on palpation of her right lower extremity. Her ECG is unremarkable and her lab tests show a positive D-dimer assay and no evidence of pregnancy. Given her young age, you order a V/Q scan and lower extremity ultrasound, rather than a CTA with CTV, in order to minimize her radiation exposure. The V/Q scan comes back as nondiagnostic and the lower extremity ultrasound is negative. Can acute PE be effectively ruled out in this case?

Suggested Answer:
This patient, at high clinical suspicion of acute PE, should undergo further testing to effectively rule out PE. In this study, V/Q scans and CTA had similar accuracy for detecting acute PE. However, the majority of V/Q scans (54.2%, 386/712) performed were nondiagnostic. Of these patients, 2.6% (10/386) had PE diagnosed by CTA or conventional angiography in the initial baseline diagnostic period. Therefore, those at high clinical suspicion with nondiagnostic V/Q scans should undergo CTA to effectively rule out acute PE.

References

1. Anderson DR, Kahn SR, Rodger MA, et al. Computed tomographic pulmonary angiography vs ventilation-perfusion lung scanning in patients with suspected pulmonary embolism: a randomized controlled trial. *JAMA*. 2007;298(23):2743–2753.
2. Musset D, Parent F, Meyer G, et al. Diagnostic strategy for patients with suspected pulmonary embolism: a prospective multicentre outcome study. *Lancet*. 2002;360(9349):1914–1920.
3. Van Strijen MJ, De Monye W, Schiereck J, et al. Single-detector helical computed tomography as the primary diagnostic test in suspected pulmonary embolism: a multicenter clinical management study of 510 patients [published correction appears in *Ann Intern Med*. 2003;139(5 pt 1):387]. *Ann Intern Med*. 2003;138(4):307–314.

4. Kruip MJH, Slob MJ, Schijen JH, van der Heul C, Büller HR. Use of a clinical decision rule in combination with d-dimer concentration in diagnostic workup of patients with suspected pulmonary embolism. *Arch Intern Med.* 2002;162(14):1631–1635.

5. Wells PS, Anderson DR, Rodger M, et al. Excluding pulmonary embolism at the bedside without diagnostic imaging: management of patients with suspected pulmonary embolism presenting to the emergency department by using a simple clinical model and D-dimer. *Ann Intern Med.* 2001;135(2):98–107.

6. Fesmire FM, Brown MD, Espinosa JA, et al. Critical issues in the evaluation and management of adult patients presenting to the emergency department with suspected pulmonary embolism. *Ann Emerg Med,* 2011;57(6):628–652.

7. Bettman MA, Baginski SG, White RD, et al. ACR appropriateness criteria acute chest pain—suspected pulmonary embolism. *J Thorac Imaging.* 2012;27(2):W28–W31.

19

Screening for Coronary Artery Disease in Asymptomatic Patients with Diabetes

The DIAD Study

MICHAEL E. HOCHMAN

> The strategy of routine screening for [coronary artery disease] in patients with type 2 diabetes is based on the premise that testing could accurately identify a significant number of individuals at particularly high risk and lead to various interventions that prevent cardiac events. However, the results of the DIAD study would appear to refute this notion.
>
> —Young et al.[1]

Research Question: Should asymptomatic patients with type 2 diabetes—who are at high risk for cardiac events—be screened for coronary artery disease (CAD)?[1]

Funding: The National Institutes of Health, Bristol Myers-Squibb Medical Imaging, and Astellas Pharma.

Year Study Began: 2000

Year Study Published: 2009

Study Location: 14 centers in the United States and Canada.

Who Was Studied: Adults 50–75 years of age with type 2 diabetes.

Who Was Excluded: Patients with symptoms of angina, recent stress testing or coronary angiography, prior cardiac events, a markedly abnormal baseline electrocardiogram, or a limited life expectancy.

How Many Patients: 1,123

Study Overview: See Figure 19.1 for a summary of DIAD's design.

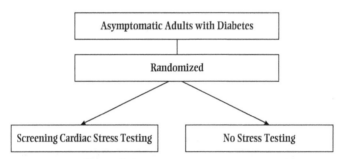

Figure 19.1 Summary of DIAD's design.

Study Intervention: Patients in the group assigned to cardiac stress testing received an adenosine-stress and radionuclide myocardial perfusion scan (see Figure 19.2). Those with abnormal stress tests were managed according to the judgment of their providers (i.e., they might be managed with medical therapy or they might receive follow-up coronary angiography and/or revascularization at their physician's discretion). Patients in the control group did not undergo stress testing unless they developed symptoms for which stress testing was indicated.

Follow-Up: Mean 4.8 years

Endpoints: Primary outcome: a composite of nonfatal myocardial infarction and cardiac death. Secondary outcomes: unstable angina, heart failure, stroke, and coronary revascularization.

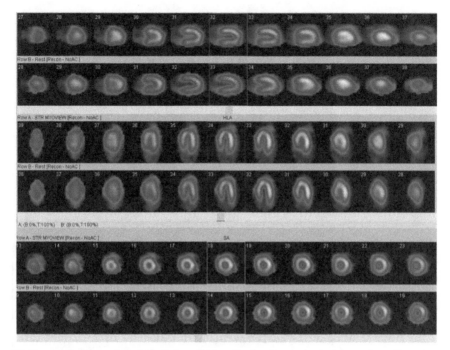

Figure 19.2 Normal myocardial perfusion single-photon emission tomography (SPECT) examination.

RESULTS

- In the screening group, 22% of patients had abnormal stress tests, including 10% who had a small perfusion defect, 6% who had a moderate or large perfusion defect, and 6% who had a nonperfusion abnormality.
- 2% of patients with normal test results and 2% with small perfusion defects had cardiac events during the study period, compared with 12.1% of patients with moderate or large perfusion defects and 6.7% with nonperfusion abnormalities.
- In the screening group, 4.4% of patients received coronary angiography within 120 days of their stress test; in comparison, 0.5% of patients in the nonscreened group received coronary angiography within 120 days of randomization.
- There were no significant differences in cardiovascular outcomes between the screened and nonscreened groups (see Table 19.1).

Table 19.1. DIAD's KEY FINDINGS

Outcome	Screening Group	Nonscreened Group	P Value
Myocardial infarction or cardiac death	2.7%	3.0%	0.73
Unstable angina	0.7%	0.5%	0.70
Heart failure	1.2%	1.2%	0.99
Stroke	1.8%	0.9%	0.20
Revascularizations	5.5%	7.8%	0.14
All-cause mortality[a]	3.2%	2.7%	0.60

[a]All-cause mortality was not a predefined endpoint.

CLINICAL CASE: SCREENING FOR CORONARY ARTERY DISEASE IN ASYMPTOMATIC PATIENTS WITH DIABETES

Case History:

You are evaluating a 52-year-old woman with diabetes in an urgent care clinic for chest pain. The pain began 3 days ago after the patient spent the afternoon with her 1-year-old grandson. During that afternoon, the woman had to lift the baby numerous times. The pain occurs on the left side of her chest and back whenever she raises her arms above her head. She does not have any pain with walking, and she denies any associated symptoms such as shortness of breath, nausea, vomiting, or diaphoresis.

You believe that this woman's chest pain is musculoskeletal in origin, and that the probability of a cardiac etiology is remote. Still, the woman is at increased cardiac risk because of her diabetes, and could be having an atypical cardiac presentation. You wonder whether or not to order a stress test for this patient. Do the results of DIAD affect your thinking?

Suggested Answer:

DIAD showed that patients with diabetes without symptoms of CAD do not appear to benefit from screening stress tests. While the woman in this vignette has chest pain, your clinical suspicion that the symptoms are due to CAD is very low. Even if you were to order a stress test and it was suggestive of CAD, it is still likely that the chest pain she is experiencing is unrelated to the stress test findings. In other words, you probably wouldn't "believe the results" if the stress test were to be positive. Thus, ordering a stress test in this woman would likely have the same impact as ordering a stress test in an asymptomatic woman with diabetes: there would be a 22% chance that the stress test would be abnormal, but knowing this information would be unlikely to aid in the patient's treatment.

Criticisms and Limitations: Cardiac event rates in the study were lower than among the general population of patients with diabetes, perhaps because (as the authors assert) the patients were well managed with aspirin, statins, and angiotensin-converting enzyme inhibitors. It is possible that screening stress tests might be beneficial among a less well-managed cohort of patients. In addition, because the event rate was lower than expected, the trial was underpowered to detect small differences between the groups.

Other Relevant Studies and Information:

- Guidelines from the American Diabetes Association do not recommend screening for coronary artery disease in asymptomatic patients with diabetes,[2] while the American College of Cardiology/ American Heart Association recommends exercise stress testing only among asymptomatic patients with diabetes who plan to begin an exercise program.[3]

Summary and Implications: Screening stress tests in patients with type 2 diabetes are abnormal 22% of the time. However, detecting these abnormalities does not appear to aid in patient management.

References

1. Young LH et al. Cardiac outcomes after screening for asymptomatic coronary artery disease in patients with type 2 diabetes: the DIAD study: a randomized controlled trial. *JAMA.* 2009;301(15):1547–1555.
2. American Diabetes Association. Standards of medical care in diabetes—2013. *Diabetes Care.* 2013;36(Suppl 1):S11.
3. Gibbons RJ et al. ACC/AHA 2002 guideline update for exercise testing: summary article: a report of the American College of Cardiology/American Heart Association Task Force on Practice Guidelines (Committee to Update the 1997 Exercise Testing Guidelines). *J Am Coll Cardiol.* 2002;40(8):1531.

20

Diagnostic Performance of CT Coronary Angiography

The CorE 64 Study

CHRISTOPH I. LEE

> . . . we found that multidetector CT angiography has a reliable accuracy for the diagnosis of obstructive coronary disease . . . However, given the positive predictive value of 91% and the negative predictive value of 83%, multidetector CT angiography cannot replace conventional coronary angiography in this population of patients at present.
>
> —MILLER ET AL.[1]

Research Question: What is the diagnostic accuracy of 64-row, 0.5-mm multidetector CT angiography compared with conventional coronary angiography in patients with suspected coronary artery disease (CAD)?

Funding: Toshiba Medical Systems, the Doris Duke Charitable Foundation, the National Heart, Lung, and Blood Institute, the National Institute on Aging, and the Donald W. Reynolds Foundation.

Year Study Began: 2005

Year Study Published: 2008

Study Location: Nine medical centers in seven countries (Brazil, Canada, Germany, Japan, Singapore, the United States, and the Netherlands).

Who Was Studied: Adult patients ≥40 years of age, suspected symptomatic CAD, and referred for conventional coronary angiography.

Who Was Excluded: Patients with Agatston calcium scores >600, history of cardiac surgery, contraindication to iodinated contrast, multiple myeloma, organ transplant, elevated serum creatinine or low creatinine clearance, atrial fibrillation, heart failure, aortic stenosis, percutaneous coronary intervention within past 6 months, beta-blocker intolerance, body mass index >40.

How Many Patients: 291

Study Overview: Prospective, multicenter, international, blinded single-arm study.

Interventions: Patients underwent CT coronary calcium scoring and multidetector CT angiography (using 64-row scanners with slice thickness of 0.5 mm) before conventional coronary angiography. Two independent observers visually assessed stenosis on images at a centralized core laboratory, and any interreader visual and quantitative differences >50% were resolved by a third observer.

Follow-Up: At 7 and 30 days after conventional coronary angiography.

Endpoints: The area under the receiver-operating-characteristic curve (AUC) was used to evaluate diagnostic accuracy of CT angiography relative to conventional angiography and subsequent revascularization status. Disease severity was evaluated using a modified Duke Coronary Artery Disease Index, with stenoses of ≥50% in any vessel greater than 1.5 mm in diameter considered obstructive CAD.

RESULTS

- After conventional coronary angiography, 56% (163/291) of patients had obstructive CAD, with stenosis of ≥50% (Figure 20.1).
- At follow-up after 30 days, 98 patients underwent percutaneous or surgical revascularization, 2 had a contrast reaction after CT angiography, 2 had myocardial infarction, 1 had a transient ischemic attack, and 1 died after coronary angioplasty.
- Patient-based diagnostic accuracy of CT angiography for detecting stenosis of ≥50% was comparable to conventional angiography with an AUC = 0.93 (95% CI, 0.90–0.96) (Table 20.1).
- CT angiography was similar to conventional angiography for identifying patients who subsequently underwent

revascularization: AUC for CT angiography = 0.84 (95% CI, 0.79–0.88) and AUC for conventional angiography = 0.82 (95% CI, 0.77–0.86).

- Vessel-based diagnostic accuracy of CT angiography was similar to conventional angiography for detecting stenosis, with an AUC = 0.91 (95% CI, 0.88–0.93), with no significant differences among individual AUCs for the right, left anterior descending, and left circumflex coronary arteries.

- CT and conventional angiography assessments of disease severity were well correlated ($r = 0.81$; 95% CI, 0.76, 0.84), with the same AUC of 0.93 ($P = 0.69$).

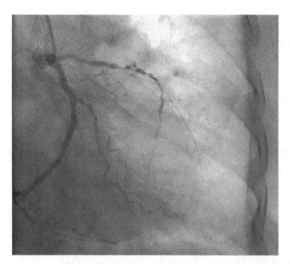

Figure 20.1 Fluoroscopic image from a cardiac catheterization with multifocal severe stenotic disease throughout the left anterior descending (LAD) coronary artery.

Table 20.1. THE TRIAL'S KEY FINDINGS

Measure of MDCTA Diagnostic Accuracy Relative to Conventional Coronary Angiography	Patient-Based Quantitative Detection by MDCTA	Patient-Based Visual Detection by MDCTA
n	291	291
False positive (no.)	13	11
False negative (no.)	24	28
Sensitivity (%, 95% CI)	85% (79%–90%)	83% (76%–88%)
Specificity (%, 95% CI)	90% (83%–94%)	91% (85%–96%)
PPV (%, 95% CI)	91% (86%–95%)	92% (87%–96%)
NPV (%, 95% CI)	83% (75%–89%)	81% (73%–87%)

MDCTA = multidetector computed tomography angiography; CI = confidence interval; PPV = positive predictive value; NPV = negative predictive value.

Criticisms and Limitations: The study population had a higher prevalence of CAD (56%) than seen in the general population. The study was not designed to test multidetector CT angiography as a replacement for conventional angiography, but only to compare its diagnostic accuracy with conventional angiography as a gold standard. Many of the exclusion criteria for this study are not necessarily criteria that would exclude other noninvasive diagnostic approaches (e.g., myocardial perfusion scintigraphy).

Other Relevant Studies and Information:

- Conventional coronary angiography, while invasive, remains the gold standard for diagnosing obstructive CAD by revealing the extent and severity of obstruction and identifying patients who may benefit from revascularization.[2,3]
- The ACCURACY (Assessment by Coronary Computed Tomographic Angiography of Individuals Undergoing Invasive Coronary Angiography) study enrolled 245 patients with chest pain referred for conventional coronary angiography at 16 US sites.[4] On a per-patient basis, sensitivity of coronary CT angiography was 94%–95%, depending on the cutpoint chosen to represent a positive invasive coronary angiogram, and specificity was 82%.
- A recent meta-analysis of 42 diagnostic accuracy studies and 11 patient outcome studies found a pooled mean sensitivity for CT angiography of 98% (95% CI, 96%–99%) and specificity of 85% (95% CI, 81%–89%) for diagnosing symptomatic CAD.[5]
- Newer-generation, prospectively gated 256- and 320-slice CT angiography increases the craniocaudal coverage and provides more stable image quality at equivalent radiation doses.[6]
- The American College of Cardiology, Society of Cardiovascular Computed Tomography, American College of Radiology, American Heart Association, American Society of Echocardiography, American Society of Nuclear Cardiology, North American Society for Cardiovascular Imaging, Society for Cardiovascular Angiography and Interventions, and Society for Cardiovascular Magnetic Resonance consider CT angiography appropriate in the following diagnostic settings: (1) evaluation of new or worsening symptoms in setting of previous normal stress imaging study, and (2) discordant ECG, exercise, and imaging results.[7]
- The American College of Radiology gives CT coronary angiography a "may be appropriate" rating (score 6 out of 9) for patients with chest pain suggestive of acute coronary syndrome, but

low-to-intermediate likelihood for CAD in the absence of cardiac enzyme elevation and ischemic ST changes.[8]

Summary and Implications: CT angiography accurately detects presence and severity of CAD in symptomatic patients with a calcium score of ≤600 and helps predict need of subsequent revascularization, but it cannot completely replace conventional coronary angigraphy at this time.

CLINICAL CASE: DIAGNOSING CORONARY ARTERY DISEASE

Case History:

A 62-year-old male is visiting your outpatient cardiology clinic for a second opinion regarding the need for conventional coronary angiography. Another physician has recommended the procedure in order to determine whether he has significant coronary artery stenosis. Due to mild recurrent chest pain, a family history of coronary artery disease, and borderline hypertension and diabetes, he obtained a CT coronary screening exam with a calcium score of 200. A recent nuclear stress imaging test was equivocal due to poor image quality, and an ECG was normal. After you conduct a physical exam and review his history, you determine that he is clinically at low-to-intermediate risk for having significant CAD. Which diagnostic test should you recommend?

Suggested Answer:

The gold standard diagnostic test for CAD remains conventional coronary angiography. However, this patient has a low CT calcium score and the CorE64 Study determined that CT angiography is accurate for detecting the presence and severity of CAD in symptomatic patients with a calcium score of ≤600. One alternative to discuss with your patient is the possibility of undergoing a noninvasive CT angiography study to provide further evidence by imaging that no significant coronary stenosis is present.

References

1. Miller JM, Rochitte CE, Dewey M, et al. Diagnostic performance of coronary angiography by 64-row CT. *NEJM*. 2008;359(22):234–236.
2. Ringqvist I, Fisher LD, Mock M, et al. Prognostic value of angiographic indices of coronary artery disease from the Coronary Artery Surgery Study (CASS). *J Clin Invest*. 1983;71(6):1854–1866.

3. Smith SCJr, Feldman TE, Hirshfeld JWJr, et al. ACC/AHA/SCAI 2005 Guideline Update for Percutaneous Coronary Intervention—summary article: a report of the American College of Cardiology/American Heart Association Task Force on Practice Guidelines (ACC/AHA/SCAI Writing Committee to Update the 2001 Guidelines for Percutaneous Coronary Intervention). *Circulation.* 2006;113(1):156–175.

4. Budoff MJ, Dowe D, Jollis JG, et al. Diagnostic performance of 64-multidetector row coronary computed tomographic angiography for evaluation of coronary artery stenosis in individuals without known coronary artery disease: results from the prospective multicenter ACCURACY (Assessment by Coronary Computed Tomographic Angiography of Individuals Undergoing Invasive Coronary Angiography) trial. *J Am Coll Cardiol.* 2008;52(21):1724–1732.

5. Ollendorf DA, Kuba M, Pearson SD. The diagnostic performance of multi-slice coronary computed tomographic angiography: a systematic review. *J Gen Intern Med.* 2011;26(3):307–316.

6. Klass O, Walker M, Siebach A, et al. Prospectively gated axial CT coronary angiography: comparison of image quality and effective radiation dose between 64- and 256-slice CT. *Eur Radiol.* 2010;20(5):1124–1131.

7. Taylor AJ, Cerqueira M, Hodgson JM, et al. ACCF/SCCT/ACR/AHA/ASE/ ASNC/NASCI/SCAI/SCMR 2010 Appropriate Use Criteria for Cardiac Computed Tomography. A Report of the American College of Cardiology Foundation Appropriate Use Criteria Task Force, the Society of Cardiovascular Computed Tomography, the American College of Radiology, the American Heart Association, the American Society of Echocardiography, the American Society of Nuclear Cardiology, the North American Society for Cardiovascular Imaging, the Society for Cardiovascular Angiography and Interventions, and the Society for Cardiovascular Magnetic Resonance. *Circulation.* 2010;122(21):e525–e555.

8. American College of Radiology. ACR appropriateness criteria: chest pain suggestive of acute coronary syndrome. http://www.acr.org/~/media/da-c4a22870304676809355ebc2a9ab47.pdf. Published 1995. Revised 2014. Accessed May 20, 2015.

21

CT Angiography for Discharge of Acute Coronary Syndrome

CHRISTOPH I. LEE

> ... a strategy in which CCTA [coronary CT angiography] is used as the first imaging test for low-to-intermediate-risk patients presenting to the emergency department with a possible acute coronary syndrome appears to allow the safe discharge of patients after a negative test.
>
> —LITT ET AL.[1]

Research Question: Can a CCTA-based strategy for patients with low risk of coronary artery disease allow the safe discharge of patients from the emergency department after a negative test?

Funding: Commonwealth of Pennsylvania Department of Health and the American College of Radiology Imaging Network Foundation.

Year Study Began: 2009

Year Study Published: 2012

Study Location: Five US medical centers.

Who Was Studied: Patients >30 years of age with signs or symptoms suggestive of possible acute coronary syndrome, ECG with no evidence of acute ischemia, and an initial Thrombolysis in Myocardial Infarction risk score of 0–2.

Who Was Excluded: Symptoms clearly noncardiac in origin, comorbidity requiring admission regardless of symptoms of acute coronary syndrome, normal CCTA or conventional angiography in previous year, or contraindication to CCTA.

How Many Patients: 1,370

Study Overview: Multicenter randomized controlled trial. Low-to-intermediate risk patients were randomly assigned, in a 2:1 ratio, to undergo CCTA or traditional care.

Interventions: Patients randomized to the CCTA group were initially evaluated with CCTA (performed with 64-slice or greater multidetector CT scanner and ECG-synchronized scanning). Patients randomized to the traditional-care group had their care, including any tests, decided by their health care provider. Decisions about admission or discharge, further testing, and treatments were determined by the clinical team in both groups.

Follow-Up: Telephone follow-up at least 30 days after presentation.

Endpoints: Primary outcome was safety, indicated by the rate of myocardial infarction and cardiac death within 30 days after presentation among patients with negative CCTA. Secondary outcomes included differing rates of discharge from the emergency department, length of hospital stay, and 30-day rates of revascularization and resource utilization.

RESULTS

- No patients with a negative CCTA examination (n = 640) died or had a myocardial infarction within 30 days of presentation (0%; 95% CI, 0%–0.57%) (Table 21.1).
- Patients in the CCTA group had higher discharge rate from the emergency department (49.6% vs. 22.7%; difference 26.8%; 95% CI, 21.4%–32.2%), shorter hospital length of stay (median 18.0 hours vs. 24.8 hours, $P < 0.001$), and higher coronary artery disease diagnosis rate (9.0% vs. 3.5%; difference 5.6%; 95% CI, 0%–11.2%).

- Within 30 days of presentation, there was no significant difference between the CCTA and traditional care groups regarding use of conventional angiography (5.1% and 4.2%, respectively; 0.9% difference, 95% CI, −4.8% to 6.6%) or revascularization rate (2.7% and 1.3%, respectively; 1.4% difference, 95% CI, −4.3% to 7.0%).
- Patients in the CCTA group were less likely than patients in the traditional care group to have negative conventional angiograms (29% versus 53%; −23.7% difference, 95% CI, −48.8% to 3.3%).

Table 21.1. THE TRIAL'S KEY FINDINGS

Cardiovascular Event within 30 Days after Presentation	CCTA-Based Strategy No. (%)	Traditional Care No. (%)	Percentage Point Difference (95% CI)
Death	0	0	0
Acute myocardial infarction	10/908 (1)	5/462 (1)	0.02 (−5.6 to 5.7)
Revascularization	24/893 (3)	6/457 (1)	1.4 (−4.3 to 7.0)

CCTA = coronary CT angiography, 95% CI = 95% confidence interval.

Criticisms and Limitations: Since myocardial infarction and death rates are very low, the study could not be powered to show between-group differences in safety (e.g., no patients died within 30 days in either group). Among patients randomly assigned to the CCTA group, 16% could not undergo the test, mostly due to elevated heart rate. Findings of coronary artery stenosis on CCTA may not have been related to presenting symptoms, as CCTA is an anatomic rather than functional test.

Other Relevant Studies and Information:

- This trial's results support the findings of previous randomized controlled trials demonstrating efficacy of CCTA for triaging patients with possible acute coronary syndrome but, for the first time, also provide the statistical power to demonstrate the safety of a CCTA-based strategy for expediting discharge of low-to-intermediate risk patients from the emergency department.[2–4]
- Acute coronary syndrome is ultimately diagnosed in 10%–15% of patients presenting to the emergency department with chest pain, even though a vast majority of these patients are admitted to the

hospital (38). This CCTA-based strategy can potentially redirect many patients to be discharged home rather than being admitted, since 50%–70% of presentations for possible acute coronary syndrome are among low-to-intermediate risk patients.[5,6]

- The American College of Cardiology and the American Heart Association consider CCTA as an appropriate test for patients presenting with possible acute coronary syndrome at intermediate risk regardless of ability to exercise and for patients at low risk if they are unable to exercise.[7]
- The American College of Radiology appropriateness criteria state that CCTA "may be appropriate" (score 6 out of 9) for low-to-intermediate likelihood of coronary artery disease, in the absence of cardiac enzyme elevation and ischemic ST changes.[8]

Summary and Implications: A negative CCTA examination can be used to safely expedite the discharge of low-to-intermediate risk patients who present to emergency department with possible acute coronary syndrome (Figures 21.1 and 21.2).

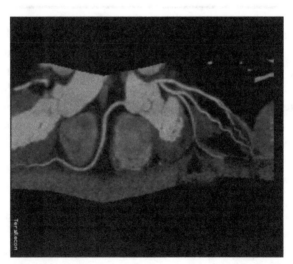

Figure 21.1 Coronary computed tomography angiography (CCTA) curved planar reformat image with normal coronary vascular anatomy. There is normal caliber and course of the coronary arteries. No atherosclerotic disease noted.

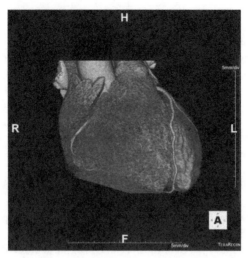

Figure 21.2 CCTA 3D volume surface render with normal coronary arteries.

CLINICAL CASE: CORONARY CT ANGIOGRAPHY FOR EARLIER DISCHARGE

Case History:
A 59-year-old male presents to the emergency department with chest tightness and pain radiating to the left upper arm. He has no history of coronary heart disease, diabetes, or hypertension. His ECG is normal with no evidence of acute ischemia. His blood pressure is 120/80 mmHg, heart rate is 104, and he weighs about 160 pounds. Would he benefit from any immediate imaging regarding a decision on whether to admit or discharge him?

Suggested Answer:
Based on the patient's history and exam findings, his Thrombosis in Myocardial Infarction score is 2, indicating a very low (2.2%) chance of 30-day mortality after a myocardial infarction. This patient would meet the inclusion criteria of this trial, which showed that a negative CCTA study could allow safe discharge home for low-to-intermediate risk patients presenting with possible acute coronary syndrome. Thus, if multislice, ECG-gated CCTA is available, then this imaging test should be pursued in the acute setting.

References

1. Litt HI, Gatsonis C, Snyder B, et al. CT angiography for safe discharge of patients with possible acute coronary syndromes. *N Engl J Med.* 2012;366(15):1393–1403.

2. Hollander JE, Chang AM, Shofer FS, McCusker CM, Baxt WG, Litt HI. Coronary computed tomographic angiography for rapid discharge of low-risk patients with potential acute coronary syndromes. *Ann Emerg Med.* 2009;53(3):295–304.

3. Hollander JE, Chang AM, Shofer FS, et al. One-year outcomes following coronary computerized tomographic angiography for evaluation of emergency department patients with potential acute coronary syndrome. *Acad Emerg Med.* 2009;16(8):693–698.

4. Hoffmann U, Bamberg F, Chae CU, et al. Coronary computed tomography angiography for early triage of patients with acute chest pain: the ROMICAT (Rule Out Myocardial Infarction using Computer Assisted Tomography) trial. *J Am Coll Cardiol.* 2009;53(18):1642–1650.

5. Selker HP, Beshansky JR, Griffith JL, et al. Use of the acute cardiac ischemia time-insensitive predictive instrument (ACI-TIPI) to assist with triage of patients with chest pain or other symptoms suggestive of acute cardiac ischemia: a multicenter, controlled clinical trial. *Ann Intern Med.* 1998;129(11):845–855.

6. Chase M, Robey JL, Zogby KE, Sease KL, Shofer FS, Hollander JE. Prospective validation of the Thrombosis in Myocardial Infarction risk score in the emergency department chest pain patient population. *Ann Emerg Med.* 2006;48(3):252–259.

7. Taylor AJ, Cerqueira M, Hodgson JM, et al. ACCF/SCCT/ACR/AHA/ASE/ ASNC/NASCI/SCAI/SCMR 2010 Appropriate Use Criteria for Cardiac Computed Tomography. A Report of the American College of Cardiology Foundation Appropriate Use Criteria Task Force, the Society of Cardiovascular Computed Tomography, the American College of Radiology, the American Heart Association, the American Society of Echocardiography, the American Society of Nuclear Cardiology, the North American Society for Cardiovascular Imaging, the Society for Cardiovascular Angiography and Interventions, and the Society for Cardiovascular Magnetic Resonance. *Circulation* 2010; 122(21):e525–55.

8. American College of Radiology. ACR appropriateness criteria: chest pain suggestive of acute coronary syndrome. http://www.acr.org/~/media/da-c4a22870304676809355ebc2a9ab47.pdf. Published 1995. Revised 2014. Accessed May 26, 2015.

22

Coronary CT Angiography in Acute Chest Pain

The Rule Out Myocardial Infarction/Ischemia Using Computed Assisted Tomography II (ROMICAT-II) Trial

CHRISTOPH I. LEE

> ... an evaluation strategy incorporating early CCTA [coronary CT angiography], as compared with a standard evaluation strategy, improved the efficiency of clinical decision making for triage in the emergency department ...
>
> —HOFFMANN ET AL.[1]

Research Question: Is evaluation incorporating CCTA more effective than standard evaluation in patients presenting to the emergency department with symptoms suggestive of acute coronary syndromes?

Funding: National Heart, Lung, and Blood Institute.

Year Study Began: 2010

Year Study Published: 2012

Study Location: Nine US hospitals.

Who Was Studied: Patients 40–74 years of age with symptoms suggestive of acute coronary syndromes, presenting with chest pain or angina of at least 5 minutes' duration within 24 hours of presentation, and no ischemic changes on ECG or positive initial troponin test.

Who Was Excluded: History of known coronary artery disease, new ischemic changes on initial ECG, initial troponin levels >99th percentile of local assay, impaired renal function, hemodynamic or clinical instability, allergy to iodinated contrast, body mass index >40, symptomatic asthma.

How Many Patients: 1,000

Study Overview: Multicenter randomized controlled trial comparing an evaluation and management strategy involving early CCTA compared with standard emergency department evaluation. All patients were included in an intention-to-treat analysis.

Interventions: Patients were randomized in a 1:1 ratio to either CCTA as part of their initial evaluation or standard evaluation, but after initial evaluation, patient care in both groups was at the discretion of treating physicians. CCTA studies were at least 64-slice and ECG-gated (retrospectively or prospectively gated).

Follow-Up: Telephone call 72 hours after discharge during initial presentation to the emergency department, and 28 days after discharge for all study patients.

Endpoints: The primary endpoint was length of stay in the hospital. Secondary endpoints included time to diagnosis of acute coronary syndrome, direct discharge rate from the emergency department, resource utilization and costs during the initial 28 days, and cumulative radiation exposure over the initial 28 days. Safety variables included undetected acute coronary syndrome and major cardiovascular events over the initial 28 days (death, myocardial infarction, unstable angina, or urgent revascularization).

RESULTS

- Patients in the early CCTA group had lower mean lengths of stay in the hospital (reduced by 7.6 hours, $P < 0.001$) and were more likely to be discharged directly from the emergency department (47% vs. 12%, $P < 0.001$) (Table 22.1 and Figure 22.1).
- Patients in the CCTA group underwent more diagnostic testing than patients in the standard evaluation group ($P < 0.001$), but there was no significant difference between groups for rate of conventional angiography and rate of coronary revascularization ($P = 0.06$ and 0.16, respectively).
- Cumulative radiation exposure was significantly higher in the CCTA group ($P < 0.001$), but patients who underwent 128-slice, dual-source CCTA had about half the radiation exposure compared to the remaining CCTA patients.
- The mean costs of care were similar between the CCTA and standard care groups ($4,289 and $4,060, respectively; $P = 0.65$).
- There were no cases of undetected acute coronary syndromes in either group, and no significant differences in major cardiac events at 28 days between groups ($P = 0.18$).

Table 22.1. THE TRIAL'S KEY FINDINGS

Endpoint	CCTA Group (n = 501)	Standard Evaluation Group (n = 499)	P value
Length of hospital stay— mean hours (interquartile ranges)	8.6 (6.4–27.6)	26.7 (21.4–30.6)	<0.001
Time to diagnosis— mean hours (interquartile ranges)	5.8 (4.0–9.0)	21.0 (8.5–23.8)	<0.001
Direct discharge home from emergency department—no. (%)	233 (47%)	62 (12%)	<0.001
Major adverse cardiovascular events at 28 days—no.	2	6	0.18

CCTA = coronary CT angiography.

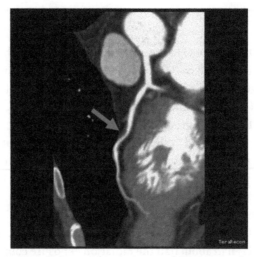

Figure 22.1 CCTA curved planar reformat image of the LAD, with multifocal stenotic disease. Note the large noncalcified plaque causing significant focal stenosis (arrow).

Criticisms and Limitations: Patient enrollment was only during weekday hours and timing of decisions to discharge or hospitalize may be different during the night. The results of this trial cannot be generalized to sites that use a dedicated accelerated diagnostic protocol (the Thrombolysis in Myocardial Infarction score with ECG and biomarker findings) as their standard evaluation. There may have been bias (due to lack of blinding) toward earlier discharge in the CCTA group. Results of the study cannot be generalized to patients <40 years and >74 years of age.

Other Relevant Studies and Information:

- ROMICAT-1 was a blinded observational study that showed a normal CCTA study had a high negative predictive value for ruling out acute coronary syndromes during the index hospitalization and major adverse cardiovascular events over the 2 subsequent years.[2]
- Two previous randomized multicenter trials demonstrated that CCTA could facilitate more efficient triage of low-risk patients for ruling out coronary artery disease compared to myocardial perfusion imaging.[3,4]
- The American College of Cardiology and the American Heart Association consider CCTA as an appropriate test for patients presenting with possible acute coronary syndrome at intermediate risk regardless of ability to exercise and for patients at low risk if they are unable to exercise.[5]

- The American College of Radiology appropriateness criteria state that CCTA "may be appropriate" (score 6 out of 9) for low-to-intermediate likelihood of coronary artery disease, in the absence of cardiac enzyme elevation and ischemic ST changes.[6]

Summary and Implications: For patients presenting to the emergency department with symptoms suggesting acute coronary syndromes, incorporating early CCTA into the triage strategy improves diagnostic efficiency, with more direct discharges from the emergency department and shorter lengths of stay for those admitted. This improved efficiency comes without greater risk for undetected acute coronary syndromes and no significant increase in costs.

CLINICAL CASE: CORONARY CT ANGIOGRAPHY FOR SHORTER LENGTH OF STAY

Case History:

A 64-year-old female presents with symptoms, including chest pain and shortness of breath, suggestive of acute coronary syndrome. There are no ischemic changes on ECG and her initial troponin tests are not >99th percentile of the local assay. Even though she is at low to intermediate risk, she is highly likely to be admitted as an inpatient based on local institution protocol. Still, would there be any benefit to obtaining any imaging at this early stage of diagnostic evaluation?

Suggested Answer:

The ROMICAT-II trial demonstrated that early CCTA imaging at the time of initial evaluation in the emergency department improved diagnostic efficiency among patients with possible acute coronary syndrome. Even for the patients who were admitted to the hospital, patients in the CCTA arm had significantly lower lengths of hospital stay without increased downstream adverse events or overall healthcare costs.

References

1. Hoffmann U, Truong QA, Schoenfeld DA, et al. Coronary CT angiography versus standard evaluation in acute chest pain. *N Engl J Med.* 2012;367(4):299–308.
2. Hoffmann U, Bamberg F, Chae CU, et al. Coronary computed tomography angiography for early triage of patients with acute chest pain: the ROMICAT (Rule Out Myocardial Infarction using Computer Assisted Tomography) trial. *J Am Coll Cardiol.* 2009;53(18):1642–1650.

3. Goldstein JA, Chinnaiyan KM, Abidov A, et al. The CT-STAT (Coronary Computed Tomographic Angiography for Systematic Triage of Acute Chest Pain Patients to Treatment) trial. *J Am Coll Cardiol.* 2011;58(14):1414–1422.

4. Litt HI, Gatsonis C, Snyder B, et al. CT angiography for safe discharge of patients with possible acute coronary syndromes. *N Engl J Med.* 2012;366(15):1393–1403.

5. Taylor AJ, Cerqueira M, Hodgson JM, et al. ACCF/SCCT/ACR/AHA/ASE/ASNC/NASCI/SCAI/SCMR 2010 Appropriate Use Criteria for Cardiac Computed Tomography. A Report of the American College of Cardiology Foundation Appropriate Use Criteria Task Force, the Society of Cardiovascular Computed Tomography, the American College of Radiology, the American Heart Association, the American Society of Echocardiography, the American Society of Nuclear Cardiology, the North American Society for Cardiovascular Imaging, the Society for Cardiovascular Angiography and Interventions, and the Society for Cardiovascular Magnetic Resonance. *Circulation.* 2010;122(21):e525–e555.

6. American College of Radiology. ACR appropriateness criteria: chest pain suggestive of acute coronary syndrome. http://www.acr.org/~/media/dac4a22870304676809355ebc2a9ab47.pdf. Published 1995. Revised 2014. Accessed May 26, 2015.

23

Coronary Artery Calcium Score and Risk Classification

CHRISTOPH I. LEE

Incorporation of an individual's CACS [coronary artery calcium score] leads to a more refined estimation of future risk of CHD [coronary heart disease] events than traditional risk factors alone.
—POLONSKY ET AL.[1]

Research Question: Does adding coronary artery calcium score (CACS) to a prediction model based on traditional risk factors improve classification of coronary heart disease (CHD) risk?

Funding: National Heart, Lung, and Blood Institute.

Year Study Began: 2000

Year Study Published: 2010

Study Location: Clinics affiliated with Columbia University, Johns Hopkins University, Northwestern University, UCLA, University of Minnesota, and Wake Forest University.

Who Was Studied: A population-based cohort of patients aged 45–84 years without known cardiovascular disease (the Multi-Ethnic Study of Atherosclerosis, MESA).

Who Was Excluded: Patients with diabetes.

How Many Patients: 5,878

Study Overview: MESA was a prospective cohort study of adult patients without known cardiovascular disease. Among MESA patients, 5-year risk estimates were calculated for incident CHD, categorized as 0%–<3%, 3%–<10%, and ≥10% using Cox proportional hazards models. Model 1 used standard Framingham risk factors: age, sex, race/ethnicity, tobacco use, systolic blood pressure, antihypertensive medication use, and high-density lipoprotein and total cholesterol levels. Model 2: same risk factors plus CACS. Net reclassification improvement and distribution of risks were calculated between the two models.

Intervention: Coronary calcium scores were determined by chest CT with either cardiac-gated electron-beam CT or multidetector CT (Figures 23.1 and 23.2). Information for traditional cardiovascular risk factors (age, blood pressure, tobacco use, cholesterol, triglycerides, plasma glucose) were measured at baseline examination.

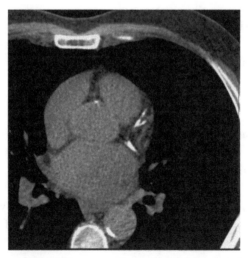

Figure 23.1 Noncontrast axial image performed for calcium scoring. Note the large coarse atherosclerotic calcifications within the proximal LAD and left circumflex (LCx) coronary arteries.

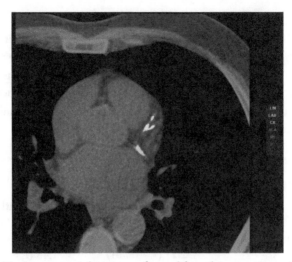

Figure 23.2 Noncontrast axial image performed for calcium scoring with color coding. Note the large coarse atherosclerotic calcifications within the proximal LAD and left circumflex (LCx) coronary arteries.

Follow-Up: Telephone interviews at 9–12 month intervals through May 2008 (patient enrolled 2000–2002). Data were abstracted for 96% of hospitalized cardiovascular events and 95% of outpatient diagnostic encounters to verify patient-reported diagnoses.

Endpoints: The main outcome measure was incident CHD events, including myocardial infarction, death due to CHD, resuscitated cardiac arrest, definite or probable angina followed by coronary revascularization, and definite angina not followed by revascularization.

RESULTS

- The prediction model was significantly improved with the inclusion of CACS, with the area under the receiver-operating-characterstic (ROC) curve for the prediction of CHD events increasing from 0.76 (95% CI, 0.72–0.79) for model 1 to 0.81 (95% CI, 0.7–0.84) for model 2 (including CACS).
- Among the entire cohort, 728 individuals were reclassified to a higher risk category, with a CHD event rate of 8.7% (95% CI, 6.9%–11.1%), and 814 individuals were reclassified to a lower risk category, with a CHD event rate of 2.7% (95% CI, 1.8%–4.1%).
- Among intermediate-risk individuals, 16% (292/1,826) were reclassified as high risk, and 39% (712/1,826) were reclassified as low risk

(net reclassification improvement, 0.55; 95% CI, 0.41–0.69; $P < 0.001$). Of the 115 CHD events among intermediate-risk individuals, 41% (48/115) occurred among individuals reclassified as high risk and 13% (15/115) occurred among individuals reclassified as low risk.

- Adding the CACS to the risk model attenuated the risk association with all of the other risk factors, suggesting the CACS has substantial influence on overall risk (see Table 23.1).

Table 23.1. RISK OF CORONARY HEART DISEASE EVENTS ASSOCIATED WITH TRADITIONAL RISK FACTORS WITHOUT AND WITH CACS

Risk Factor	Model without CACS, HR and P Value	Model with CACS, HR and P Value
Age (per 5-year increase)	1.30 ($P < 0.001$)	1.08 ($P = 0.09$)
Male	2.21 ($P < 0.001$)	1.48 ($P = 0.02$)
Systolic blood pressure (per 10-mm Hg increase)	1.10 ($P = 0.003$)	1.08 ($P = 0.03$)
Antihypertensive use	1.61 ($P = 0.001$)	1.37 ($P = 0.03$)
Total cholesterol (per 10 mg/dL increase)	1.07 ($P = 0.001$)	1.05 ($P = 0.01$)
High density lipoprotein cholesterol (per 10 mg/dL increase)	0.81 ($P < 0.001$)	0.84 ($P = 0.002$)
Current smoker	1.91 ($P = 0.003$)	1.54 ($P = 0.05$)
CACS	–	1.41 ($P < 0.001$)

CACS = coronary artery calcium score; HR = hazard ratio.

Criticisms and Limitations: A relatively smaller proportion of the MESA population was reclassified as high risk (5.1%) than seen in the general population. A longer follow-up period may have led to additional CHD events not captured by this analysis. Both treating physicians and patients were informed of the CACS, which may have led to biases for diagnosing angina or more intensive risk factor modification. This study did not address whether screening for subclinical disease with CACS actually leads to improved patient outcomes.

Other Relevant Studies and Information:

- Previous analysis of data from the MESA study found that CACS >300 was associated with a hazard ratio of nearly 10 for future CHD events.[2]
- Since only 4 of >3,000 low-risk individuals were reclassified as high risk after researchers added CACS to the risk model, CACS may not be an efficient screening method for low-risk individuals.

- For a new risk biomarker (e.g., CACS), the concept of net reclassification improvement measures the extent to which individuals with or without the biomarker are appropriately reclassified into clinically accepted lower or higher risk categories after its addition to a traditional risk model.[3,4]
- The American College of Cardiology, American Heart Association, and the American College of Radiology consider the use of noncontrast CT to determine CACS to help estimate risk among intermediate-risk individuals as appropriate (score 7 out of 9) and inappropriate (score 2 of 9) in low-risk individuals. They also consider CACS as appropriate (score 7 of 9) for individuals with a family history of premature CAD.[5,6]

Summary and Implications: Adding CACS to traditional risk factors produces significant improvements in classification of patients for future risk of CHD events. This is especially true for intermediate-risk individuals who stand to benefit the most from a CACS-adjusted risk stratification strategy, as the majority of these individuals will be reclassified as low or high risk, where treatment strategies are better established.

CLINICAL CASE: PREDICTING RISK WITH CT CORONARY ARTERY CALCIUM SCORES

Case History:
A 52-year-old male presents to your primary care clinic for an annual physical examination and preventive medicine check-up. He has a family history of coronary heart disease, but reports no chest pain symptoms. After asking him about his smoking history, taking his blood pressure, reviewing his medication list, and reviewing his laboratory results, you determine that he is at intermediate 5-year risk of an adverse CHD-related event. Would imaging be helpful in this situation?

Suggested Answer:
Based on the findings of this study, this patient may benefit from noncontrast chest CT to determine a CACS. This additional information could help further stratify this intermediate-risk patient to a higher risk classification, and make him eligible to receive more intensive therapy as a result of screening. These potential preventive interventions may include lifestyle changes, mini dose aspirin, starting a statin, and/or treating hypertension.

References

1. Polonsky TS, McClelland RL, Jorgensen NW, et al. Coronary artery calcium score and risk classification for coronary heart disease prediction. *JAMA*. 2010;303(16):1610–1616.
2. Detrano R, Guerci AD, Carr JJ, et al. Coronary calcium as a predictor of coronary events in four racial or ethnic groups. *N Engl J Med*. 2008;358(13):1336–1345.
3. Pencina MJ, D'Agostino RBSr, D'Agostino RBJr, Vasan RS. Evaluating the added predictive ability of a new marker: from area under the ROC curve to reclassification and beyond. *Stat Med*. 2008;27(2):157–172.
4. Tzoulaki I, Liberopoulos G, Ioannidis JP. Assessment of claims of improved prediction beyond the Framingham risk score. *JAMA*. 2009;302(21):2345–2352.
5. Taylor AJ, Cerqueira M, Hodgson JM, et al. ACCF/SCCT/ACR/AHA/ASE/ ASNC/NASCI/SCAI/SCMR 2010 Appropriate Use Criteria for Cardiac Computed Tomography. A Report of the American College of Cardiology Foundation Appropriate Use Criteria Task Force, the Society of Cardiovascular Computed Tomography, the American College of Radiology, the American Heart Association, the American Society of Echocardiography, the American Society of Nuclear Cardiology, the North American Society for Cardiovascular Imaging, the Society for Cardiovascular Angiography and Interventions, and the Society for Cardiovascular Magnetic Resonance. *Circulation*. 2010;122(21):e525–e555.
6. American College of Radiology. ACR appropriateness criteria: asymptomatic patient at risk for coronary artery disease. https://acsearch.acr.org/docs/3082570/ Narrative/. Published 2013. Accessed May 26, 2015.

Abdominal and Pelvic Pain

24

Abdominal Aortic Aneurysm Screening

The Multicentre Aneurysm Screening Study (MASS)

CHRISTOPH I. LEE

> Our findings indicate that screening can significantly reduce mortality
> rates associated with abdominal aortic aneurysms . . .
>
> —ASHTON ET AL.[1]

Research Question: Does ultrasound screening for abdominal aortic aneurysm (AAA) decrease mortality?

Funding: UK Medical Research Council and the Department of Health.

Year Study Began: 1997

Year Study Published: 2002

Study Location: Four UK medical centers (Portsmouth, Southampton, Winchester, Oxford).

Who Was Studied: Men aged 65–74 years identified from Health Authority and family doctor patient lists.

Who Was Excluded: Men identified by their family doctor as being terminally ill, having serious comorbidities, or having undergone a previous AAA repair.

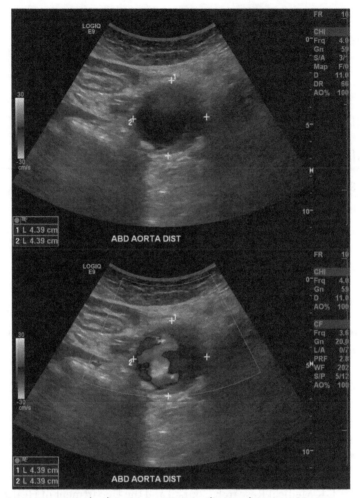

Figure 24.1 Grayscale (top) and color Doppler (bottom) transverse ultrasound images of a large abdominal aortic aneurysm. Note the mural thrombus.

How Many Patients: 67,800

Study Overview: Randomized controlled trial. Patients were randomly assigned to either receive an invitation for a screening abdominal ultrasound (invited group) or not (control group). Men with normal aortas (<3 cm diameter) and those where the aorta was not visualized were not rescanned. Patients with aortas measuring 3.0–4.4 cm in diameter were rescanned annually, while patients with aortas measuring 4.5–5.4 cm were rescanned at 3-month intervals. Urgent referral to surgery was recommended for patients with aortas measuring

≥5.5 cm in diameter, and those with growth of ≥1 cm per year. An intention-to-treat analysis based on cause of death was performed. Quality of life was assessed using four standardized scales among screened and nonscreened study participants.

Exposure: Screening ultrasounds were performed by experienced sonographers using a portable ultrasound machine. The maximum transverse and anterior-posterior diameters of the abdominal aorta were measured and recorded (Figure 24.1).

Follow-Up: Mean of 4.1 years follow-up for men with AAA ≥3 cm in diameter.

Endpoints: Primary outcome was mortality related to AAA. Secondary outcomes included all-cause mortality, frequency of ruptured AAA, and effect of screening and surgery on quality of life.

RESULTS

- 80% (27,147/33,839) of men invited accepted the invitation to screen, with 1,333 (4.9% of those scanned) having AAAs detected.
- The invited group had 65 aneurysm-related deaths (0.19% absolute risk) and the control group had 113 aneurysm-related deaths (0.33% absolute risk) (Table 24.1).
- The risk reduction was 42% for those invited to screen (95% CI, 22%–58%) and 53% for those who attended screening (95% CI, 30%–64%) compared to the control group.
- The overall 30-day mortality rate was 6% (24/414) after elective surgery and 37% (30/81) after emergency surgery for aneurysm. While the invited group had fewer emergency operations than the control group (27 vs. 54), the overall 30-day mortality rate did not differ between groups ($P = 0.32$).
- There was no statistically significant difference in all-cause mortality between the two groups.
- There were no differences in anxiety or depression scores 6 weeks after screening between those screened negative and those screened positive.
- There were no differences in mood, physical or mental scores, or weighted health index scores between groups 12 months after screening or surgery, with slightly higher heath ratings for those who underwent surgery.

Table 24.1. THE TRIAL'S KEY FINDINGS

Outcome Measure	Control Group (n = 33,961)	Invited Group (n = 33,839)
Deaths from ruptured AAA	91	37
Deaths from ruptured aortic aneurysm (site unspecified)	13	13
AAA-related death rate (per 1,000 person-years) (95% CI)	0.85 (0.71–1.02)[a]	0.49 (0.39–0.63)[a]
Nonfatal ruptured AAA rate (per 1,000 person-years) (95% CI)	1.06 (0.89–1.25)[b]	0.62 (0.50–0.77)[b]

AAA = abdominal aortic aneurysm; 95% CI = 95% confidence interval.
[a]Hazard ratio for invited group, with control group as reference, was 0.58 (95% CI, 0.42–0.78; $P = 0.0002$).
[b]Hazard ratio for invited group, with control group as reference, was 0.59 (95% CI, 0.45–0.77; $P = 0.00006$).

Criticisms and Limitations: The portable ultrasound machine used in this study represents outdated technology. A small proportion of patients' aortas (about 1%) were not visualized on ultrasound, and these patients were not re-screened. The ICD-9 codes for aortic aneurysms, in addition to codes for AAAs, may have led to the inclusion of patients with thoracic aneurysms undetectable on abdominal ultrasound, biasing results against screening.

Other Relevant Studies and Information:

- There is a six times greater prevalence of AAA-related deaths among men than women[2]; thus, routine screening is currently only recommended for men.
- At 10-year follow-up, screening men 65–74 years old for AAA through the MASS study showed persistent mortality benefit and more favorable cost-effectiveness over time.[3]
- AAAs are more prevalent among individuals who have ever smoked, and simulation modeling suggests inviting only men aged 65–74 years with a history of ever smoking (accounting for 69% of men in this age group) would account for 89% of the anticipated mortality reduction.[4]
- The US Preventive Services Task Force currently recommends one-time ultrasound screening for AAA in men ages 65–75 years old who have ever smoked (B recommendation) and that clinicians selectively

offer screening in men ages 65–75 years old who have never smoked (C recommendation).[5]

- In 2009, the Society for Vascular Surgery issued guidelines recommending screening ultrasound for men >65 years (and >55 years if a family history of AAA) and for women >65 years who smoked or have a family history (citing a higher aneurysm rupture rate among women).[6]

Summary and Implications: Screening for AAAs can decrease aneurysm-related mortality rates. However, since AAAs contribute to <3% of all deaths, there is no significant decrease in all-cause mortality from screening. This trial further found no adverse effects on emotional states of patients who underwent screening or subsequent surgery 1 year after screening or surgery.

CLINICAL CASE: SCREENING FOR ABDOMINAL AORTIC ANEURYSM

Case History:
A 66-year-old female presents to your primary care clinic asking about screening for AAA. She smoked during her 40s and her father passed away from a ruptured AAA in his 60s. She would also like to know if a screening study would be covered by her Medicare insurance. How should you advise this patient?

Suggested Answer:
The USPSTF currently advises against screening women who have never smoked, but concluded that evidence is insufficient to assess the benefits and harms of screening women ages 65–75 years who have ever smoked. You should inform her that there may be some potential benefit from detecting an aneurysm by ultrasound, but that there is not enough evidence to suggest that the risks outweigh the potential benefits. If she chooses to undergo screening, Medicare does cover a one-time ultrasound screening study for female recipients with a family history of AAA.

References

1. Ashton HA, Buxton MJ, Day NE, et al. The Multicentre Aneurysm Screening Study (MASS) into the effects of screening on mortality in men: a randomised controlled trial. *Lancet.* 2002;360(9345):1531–1539.

2. Vardulaki KA, Walker NM, Day NE, Duffy SW, Ashton HA, Scott RAP. Quantifying the risks of hypertension age, sex and smoking in patients with abdominal aortic aneurysm. *Br J Surg.* 2000;87(2):195–200.

3. Thompson SG, Ashton HA, Gao L, Scott RA; Multicentre Aneurysm Screening Study Group. Screening men for abdominal aortic aneurysm: 10 year mortality and cost effectiveness results from the randomized Multicentre Aneurysm Screening Study. *BMJ.* 2009;338:b2307.

4. Fleming C, Whitlock EP, Beil TL, Lederle FA. Screening for abdominal aortic aneurysm: a best-evidence systematic review for the U.S. Preventive Services Task Force. *Ann Intern Med.* 2005;142(3):203–211.

5. LeFevre ML; US Preventive Services Task Force. Screening for abdominal aortic aneurysm: U.S. Preventive Services Task Force recommendation statement. *Ann Intern Med.* 2014;161(4):281–290.

6. Chaikof EL, Brewster DC, Dalman RL, et al. The care of patients with abdominal aortic aneurysm: the Society for Vascular Surgery practice guidelines. *J Vasc Surg.* 2009;50(4 Suppl):S2–S49.

25

Imaging Appendicitis in Children

CHRISTOPH I. LEE

> The addition of CTRC [CT with rectal contrast] after a negative ultra-sonography result increased the imaging sensitivity [for appendicitis] from 44% to 94%.
> —GARCIA PEÑA ET AL.[1]

Research Question: What is the accuracy of ultrasound and limited CT with rectal contrast in diagnostic pediatric appendicitis?

Funding: None reported.

Year Study Began: 1998

Year Study Published: 1999

Study Location: Single large urban pediatric teaching hospital.

Who Was Studied: Children and adolescents aged 3–21 years with equivocal findings for acute appendicitis.

Who Was Excluded: Pregnant patients, patients with previous appendectomy, or contraindication to rectal contrast.

How Many Patients: 139

Study Overview: Prospective cohort study. All children with suspected appendicitis were evaluated by a senior surgical resident under the supervision of an attending pediatric surgeon. Patients with equivocal findings were initially evaluated with pelvic ultrasound. If the ultrasound was definitive, laparotomy was performed. If the ultrasound was negative or inconclusive (e.g., appendix not visualized), then limited CT with rectal contrast of the pelvis was performed.

Exposure: Pelvic ultrasounds were performed by a pediatric radiology fellow or attending using a 5.0 and/or 7.5 MHz linear array transducer. CT with rectal contrast was performed with helical technique, limited scanning, and after rectal contrast was placed via a rectal cathether. No oral or intravenous contrast was used. Diagnosis of appendicitis was based on detecting a fluid-filed, distended tubular structure measuring at least 6 mm in diameter and/or periappendiceal inflammatory changes.

Follow-Up: All children who did not undergo surgery were contacted for follow-up at 2 weeks by telephone. Medical records of all patients were reviewed 4–6 months after study completion.

Endpoints: Sensitivity, specificity, positive predictive value, negative predictive value, and accuracy of ultrasound-CT with rectal contrast. Surgeons also estimated likelihood of appendicitis on a 1–10 scale and case management plans before imaging, after ultrasound, and after CT.

RESULTS

- Among 177 children evaluated for appendicitis during the 6-month study period, 2.3% (4/177) of patients were discharged without imaging, 19.2% (34/177) went directly to surgery without imaging, and 78.5% (139/177) underwent diagnostic imaging for clinically equivocal findings (this latter group comprised the study cohort) (Table 25.1).
- Ultrasound identified a normal appendix in 2.4% (2/83) of patients without appendicitis, while limited CT with rectal contrast identified a normal appendix in 84% (62/74) of patients without appendicitis.

- Positive findings on ultrasound or CT influenced surgeons' estimated likelihood of appendicitis ($P = 0.001$ and $P < 0.001$, respectively).
- Negative ultrasound findings did not change the surgeons' clinical confidence in ruling out appendicitis ($P = 0.06$), but negative CT findings did increase the surgeons' confidence level ($P < 0.001$).
- Ultrasound correctly changed management plans in 18.7% (26/139) of patients, while limited CT with rectal contrast correctly changed management plans in 73.1% (79/108) of patients.

Table 25.1. THE TRIAL'S KEY FINDINGS

Imaging for Appendicitis	Sensitivity	Specificity	PPV	NPV	Accuracy
Ultrasound	44%	93%	79%	75%	76%
CT after negative or equivocal ultrasound	97%	94%	85%	99%	94%
Ultrasound-CT study protocol	94%	94%	90%	97%	94%

PPV = positive predictive value; NPV = negative predictive value.

Criticisms and Limitations: This study was performed at a single academic institution; thus, its findings may not be widely generalizable. The true performance characteristics for limited CT with rectal contrast cannot be determined from this study, as CT was performed only following a negative or indeterminate ultrasound. Radiologists performing ultrasounds were aware of the surgeon's estimated likelihood of appendicitis, potentially biasing their interpretations of ultrasound examinations. Radiologists interpreting CT scans may have been the same persons who performed the ultrasounds, thus potentially biasing the interpretation of the CT scans.

Other Relevant Studies and Information:

- Ultrasound may diagnose appendicitis in a substantial proportion of pediatric patients with equivocal clinical findings without the need for radiation. For the pediatric patient population with a low pretest probability of appendicitis, ultrasound remains the primary diagnostic modality.

- For children with equivocal clinical findings, the American College of Radiology recommends beginning with ultrasound (appropriateness rating of 8 out of 9).[2] A normal appendix must be seen to reliably exclude appendicitis in patients with persistent symptoms. If the appendix is not visualized or the ultrasound is nondiagnostic, CT scan with contrast should be considered (appropriateness rating of 7 out of 9).[2]
- If CT is performed in children with equivocal findings, most experts now recommend contrast-enhanced CT rather than CT without contrast, and intravenous contrast is preferred over oral or rectal contrast.[2-4]
- Some institutions are able to offer MRI as a primary diagnostic tool for appendicitis in children with relatively high sensitivity and specificity using an abbreviated scanning protocol with the need for contrast or sedation.[5]

Summary and Implications: CT with contrast after a negative or indeterminate pelvic ultrasound leads to very high accuracy in diagnosing acute appendicitis in children (Figure 25.1).

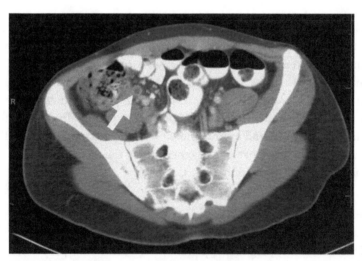

Figure 25.1 Contrast-enhanced axial CT image of the pelvis status post rectal contrast administration with acute appendicitis (arrow).

CLINICAL CASE: APPENDICITIS IN CHILDREN

Case History:

A 3-year-old male presents to the pediatric emergency department with abdominal pain and nausea. The patient has an elevated white blood cell count and the parents report that their son has not had an appetite all day. You order an ultrasound of the right lower quadrant, and the pediatric radiologists reports that the appendix was not visualized and there was no evidence of abscess or fluid collections in the right lower quadrant. What should you do next?

Suggested Answer:

Based on this study, contrast-enhanced CT should be considered in cases with equivocal ultrasound findings. This patient has signs and symptoms suspicious of appendicitis. Since the appendix was not visualized, you should order a CT with intravenous contrast. The use of additional oral or rectal contrast is institution dependent, and, in many cases, intravenous contrast alone should be sufficient for obtaining a very high accuracy for diagnosing pediatric acute appendicitis.

References

1. Garcia Peña BM, Mandl KD, Kraus SJ, et al. Ultrasonography and limited computed tomography in the diagnosis and management of appendicitis in children. *JAMA*. 1999;282:1041–1046.
2. Rosen MP, Ding A, Blake MA, et al. ACR Appropriateness Criteria right lower quadrant pain—suspected appendicitis. *J Am Coll Radiol*. 2011;8(11):749–755.
3. Anderson SW, Soto JA, Lucey BC, et al. Abdominal 64-MDCT for suspected appendicitis: the use of oral and IV contrast material versus IV contrast material only. *AJR Am J Roentgenol*. 2009;193(5):1282–1288.
4. Kepner AM, Bacasnot JV, Stalman BA. Intravenous contrast alone vs intravenous and oral contrast computed tomography for the diagnosis of appendicitis in adult ED patients. *Am J Emerg Med*. 2012;30(9):1765–1773.
5. Kulaylat AN, Moore MM, Engbrecht BW, et al. An implemented MRI program to eliminate radiation from the evaluation of pediatric appendicitis. *J Pediatr Surg*. 2015;50(8):1359–1363.

26

Low-Dose CT for Suspected Appendicitis in Young Adults

CHRISTOPH I. LEE

> Overall, our results indicate that low-dose CT, despite its limitations, may be used instead of standard-dose CT as the first line imaging test . . .
> —KIM ET AL.[1]

Research Question: Is low-dose CT just as good as standard-dose CT for diagnosing acute appendicitis in young adults?

Funding: GE Healthcare, National Research Foundation of Korea.

Year Study Began: 2009

Year Study Published: 2012

Study Location: Seoul National University Bundang Hospital, South Korea.

Who Was Studied: Young adults aged 15–44 years suspected of having appendicitis and referred for abdominal CT from the emergency department.

Who Was Excluded: Patients meeting inclusion criteria but with body mass index <18.5 kg/m^2 (ultrasound is preferred), prior cross-sectional imaging to evaluate presenting symptoms or signs, history of appendectomy, contraindication to intravenous contrast.

How Many Patients: 891

Study Overview: Single-center single-blind noninferiority randomized trial. Patients were randomized in a 1:1 ratio to undergo either low-dose or standard-dose CT of the abdomen. Care providers were not blinded to the intervention group, but patients and outcomes assessors were blinded to assignments. Radiologists of variable levels of expertise (attendings, fellows, residents) interpreted CT images and were not blinded to clinical and laboratory findings. An intention-to-treat analysis was conducted.

Interventions: All CT scans were obtained using a 16-, 64-, or 256-detector row CT scanner and with intravenous contrast. The reference tube current-time product was set to aim for an effective dose of 2 mSv in the low-dose CT group and 8 mSv in the standard-dose CT group. Experimental low-dose CT group had an actual median dose-length product of 116 mGy-cm. The standard-dose CT group had an actual median dose-length product of 521 mGy-cm. Routine 5-mm-thick images were augmented with 2-mm thin-slice images and multiplanar sliding-slab averaging techniques.

Follow-Up: Pathological examination after surgery, or review of medical records and telephone interviews 3 months after patients' initial presentation if no surgery.

Endpoints: Primary endpoint was percentage of negative appendectomies among all nonincidental appendectomies, with a noninferiority margin of 5.5 percentage points. Secondary clinical endpoints included rate of perforated appendices, proportion of patients requiring additional imaging (e.g., ultrasound or standard-dose CT performed within 7 days after initial CT examination), interval between CT acquisition and surgery or discharge, and length of hospital stay if appendectomy. Secondary diagnostic performance endpoints included area under the ROC curve (AUC), sensitivity and specificity (with grade 3 or higher on 5-point Likert scale considered to be positive for appendicitis), and diagnostic confidence (i.e., likelihood of appendicitis).

RESULTS

- In terms of negative appendectomy rate, the low-dose CT group (3.5%, 6/172) was noninferior to the standard-dose CT group (3.2%, 6/186) (difference, 0.3 percentage points; 95% CI, –3.8 to 4.6) (Table 26.1).

- In terms of appendiceal perforation rate, the low-dose CT group (26.5%, 44/166) and the standard-dose CT group (23.3%, 42/180) did not differ significantly ($P = 0.46$).
- The proportion of patients who needed additional imaging tests did not differ significantly between the low-dose CT group (3.2%, 14/438) and the standard-dose CT group (1.6%, 7/441) ($P = 0.09$).
- For diagnosis of appendicitis, the AUC for the low-dose CT group (0.970) did not differ significantly from the AUC (0.975) for the standard-dose CT group ($P = 0.69$).

Table 26.1. THE TRIAL'S KEY FINDINGS

Clinical Outcome	Low-Dose CT Group	Standard-Dose CT Group	Difference (95% CI)[a] and/or P value[b]
Negative appendectomy rate	3.5% (6/172)	3.2% (6/186)	0.3 (−3.8 to 4.6)
Appendiceal perforation rate	26.5% (44/166)	23.3% (42/180)	3.2 (−5.9 to 12.4), $P = 0.46$
Need for additional imaging	3.2% (14/438)	1.6% (7/441)	1.6 (−0.4 to 3.9), $P = 0.09$
Interval between CT and appendectomy (median hours, interquartile range)	7.1 (4.3–11.7)	5.6 (3.4–9.2)	$P = 0.02$
Interval between CT and discharge without surgery (median hours, interquartile range)	2.5 (1.5–4.2)	2.4 (1.4–4.4)	$P = 0.63$
Hospital stay associated with appendectomy (median days, interquartile range)	3.4 (2.7–4.1)	3.2 (2.5–4.1)	$P = 0.54$

[a] Percentage points.
[b] P values based on Fisher's exact test or Mann-Whitney U test. 95% CI = 95% confidence interval.

Criticisms and Limitations: Investigators experienced in and favoring low-dose CT techniques played a major role in caring for study patients, potentially introducing bias. This study was not powered to analyze potential patient-level or radiologist-level factors that may influence differential outcomes between low-dose CT and standard-dose CT groups. Only a few obese patients were involved in this study, limiting the generalizability of these results to nonobese patients.

Other Relevant Studies and Information:

- Young adults are at increased risk of radiation-induced cancer, with one study estimating that 1 in 500 women and 1 in 660 men may develop cancer during their lifetime from a single abdominal CT scan performed at the age of 20.[2]
- This study corroborates findings from several earlier exploratory studies that demonstrated that reducing CT dose by 50%–80% did not decrease accuracy for diagnosing appendicitis.[3–5]
- A multi-institutional, randomized trial comparing low-dose versus standard-dose abdominal CT among adolescents and young adults with suspected appendicitis is currently ongoing (the LOCAT trial).[6]
- The American College of Radiology considers CT abdomen and pelvis with contrast to be the most appropriate imaging examination (rating 8 out of 9) for adults and adolescents presenting with signs and symptoms suggestive of appendicitis. Ultrasound with graded compression may also be appropriate (rating 6 out of 9) in this setting.[7]

Summary and Implications: Low-dose CT is not inferior to standard-dose CT with respect to negative appendectomy rates among young adults presenting with suspected appendicitis (Figure 26.1). If used as the first-line imaging

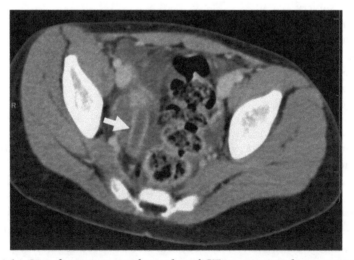

Figure 26.1 Low-dose contrast-enhanced axial CT image in a pediatric patient with acute appendicitis (arrow). Note the surrounding free fluid within the pelvis.

study in a common indication for CT, potential radiation-induced cancer risks can be reduced among this radiosensitive patient population.

CLINICAL CASE: SUSPECTED APPENDICITIS IN YOUNG ADULT

Case History:

A 24-year-old female presents to the emergency department with fever and abdominal pain that has localized to the right lower quadrant. She denies any nausea or vomiting, and has had prior episodes of generalized lower abdominal pain that have resolved and that she associates with her menstrual cycle. Her pregnancy test is negative. The patient is concerned about radiation risks from medical imaging. What are this patient's potential options for diagnostic imaging?

Suggested Answer:

Based on this study, if a low-dose CT technique is available at your institution, this patient could have her diagnostic workup for appendicitis performed with CT using the lower radiation dose. Compared to standard-dose CT, low-dose CT is not inferior with regard to negative appendectomy rates. In addition, if the patient is of thin build, you may consider starting with ultrasound with graded compression. If the appendix is visualized under ultrasound, a diagnosis may be possible without the use of any ionizing radiation to the patient.

References

1. Kim K, Kim YH, Kim SY, et al. Low-dose abdominal CT for evaluating suspected appendicitis. *N Engl J Med.* 2012; 366(17):1596–1605.
2. Smith-Bindman R, Lipson J, Marcus R, et al. Radiation dose associated with common computed tomography examinations and the associated lifetime attributable risk of cancer. *Arch Intern Med.* 2009;169(22):2078–2086.
3. Kim SY, Lee KH, Kim K, et al. Acute appendicitis in young adults: low- versus standard-radiation-dose contrast-enhanced abdominal CT for diagnosis. *Radiology.* 2011;260(2):437–45.
4. Keyzer C, Tack D, de Maertelaer V, Bohy P, Gevenois PA, Van Gansbeke D. Acute appendicitis: comparison of low-dose and standard-dose unenhanced multidetector row CT. *Radiology.* 2004;232(1):164–172.
5. Seo H, Lee KH, Kim HJ, et al. Diagnosis of acute appendicitis with sliding slab ray-sum interpretation of low-dose unenhanced CT and standard-dose i.v. contrast enhanced CT scans. *AJR Am J Roentgenol.* 2009;193(1):96–105.

6. Ahn S; LOCAT group. LOCAT (low-dose computed tomography for appendicitis trial) comparing clinical outcomes following low- vs standard-dose computed tomography as the first-line imaging test in adolescents and young adults with suspected acute appendicitis: study protocol for a randomized controlled trial. *Trials.* 2014;15:28. doi:10.1186/1745-6215-15-28.
7. Rosen MP, Ding A, Blake MA, et al. ACR Appropriateness Criteria right lower quadrant pain—suspected appendicitis. *J Am Coll Radiol.* 2011;8(11):749–755.

27

Multidetector CT for Acute Appendicitis in Adults

CHRISTOPH I. LEE

MDCT [multidetector computed tomography] can efficiently and effectively identify the approximately one quarter of patients with actual appendicitis who need urgent surgery, and it can often identify a probable alternative cause of symptoms in those who do not have appendicitis.

—PICKHARDT ET AL.[1]

Research Question: What is the diagnostic accuracy of MDCT for suspected appendicitis in adults?

Funding: None reported.

Year Study Began: 2000

Year Study Published: 2011

Study Location: Single US academic medical center.

Who Was Studied: Adult patients ≥18 years referred from the emergency department or urgent care setting to have MDCT for signs and symptoms concerning for appendicitis between years 2000–2009; MDCT performed within 24-48 hours of acute presentation.

Who Was Excluded: Patients referred for MDCT due to abdominal pain not suggestive of appendicitis (e.g., generalized pain, left-sided abdominal pain, presumed urolithiasis).

How Many Patients: 2,871

Study Overview: Retrospective cohort analysis of MDCT findings and clinical outcomes of adult patients with suspected appendicitis. Diagnostic performance of MDCT was based on the original MDCT evaluation at time of presentation interpreted by board-certified staff radiologists.

Exposure: Standard MDCT protocol included general, nonfocused imaging of the abdomen and pelvis with both oral and intravenous contrast administration. Scanners used were 4-, 8-, 16-, and 64-detector row MDCT scanners. Standard 5 mm sections, with thinner images reconstructed as needed.

Follow-Up: Minimum 12-month clinical follow-up via medical records for nonsurgical cohort.

Endpoints: Posttest assessment of MDCT interpretation for diagnosing acute appendicitis, using a reference standard of final combined clinical, surgical, and pathology findings. Diagnostic performance characteristics included sensitivity, specificity, and predictive values.

RESULTS

- 23.5% (675/2871) of the study cohort had confirmed acute appendicitis (Table 27.1).
- The positive likelihood ratio (51.3; 95% CI, 38.1–69.0) and negative likelihood ratio (0.015; 95% CI, 0.008–0.028) suggest that MDCT findings have a dominant influence on clinical management of patients suspected to have appendicitis and on posttest probabilities (Figure 27.1).
- The overall rate of negative findings at appendectomy would have decreased from 7.5% (54/716) to 4.1% (28/690) had the true-negative findings on MDCT been heeded and surgery avoided.
- MDCT helped identify an alternative diagnosis for acute abdominal pain in 42.1% (893/2,122) of patients without appendicitis or appendectomy.
- The annual appendiceal perforation rate progressively decreased from 28.9% in 2000 to 11.5% in 2009, which was inversely

proportional to MDCT volume, which increased from 138 in 2000 to 433 in 2009 for suspected cases of appendicitis.

Table 27.1. THE TRIAL'S KEY FINDINGS

MDCT Performance Characteristic	Value (95% CI)	Patients (n/N)
Sensitivity	98.5% (97.3%–99.2%)	665/675
Specificity	98.0% (97.4%–98.6%)	2,153/2,196
Negative predictive value	99.5% (99.2%–99.8%)	2,153/2,163
Positive predictive value	93.9% (91.9%–95.5%)	665/708

MDCT = multidetector computed tomography; CI = confidence interval.

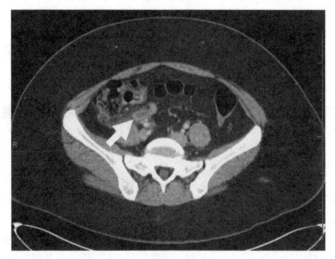

Figure 27.1 Contrast-enhanced axial CT image in an adult patient with acute appendicitis (arrow). Note the associated adjacent mesenteric fat stranding.

Criticisms and Limitations: Since some patients with equivocal clinical findings may not have been referred for MDCT, referral bias may have occurred. There was no control group in this study that did not undergo imaging evaluation. This study was performed at one academic institution and its results may not be generalizable to other settings.

Other Relevant Studies and Information:

- Routine CT use for suspected appendicitis among adults has been shown to improve patient care, reduce the use of hospital resources, and decrease overall costs.[2]

- The use of nonfocused MDCT with both oral and intravenous contrast in adults may provide the best overall sensitivity and specificity for appendicitis compared to other CT protocols (e.g., limited CT with rectal contrast), while also providing a higher yield for alternative diagnoses (which are more common than appendicitis).[1,3]
- The American College of Radiology considers CT abdomen and pelvis with contrast to be the most appropriate imaging examination (rating 8 out of 9) for adults presenting with signs and symptoms suggestive of appendicitis. Ultrasound with graded compression may also be appropriate (rating 6 out of 9) in this setting.[4]

Summary and Implications: Nonfocused abdominal MDCT is highly sensitive and specific for acute appendicitis. When incorporated into routine diagnostic algorithms, it can reduce rates of perforation and negative findings at appendectomy, and can redirect management for patients with alternative diagnoses.

CLINICAL CASE: ADULT APPENDICITIS

Case History:
A 44-year-old male presents to the emergency department with lower abdominal pain, nausea, and fever. His past medical history is significant for prior nephrolithiasis and diverticulitis, for which the patient has been treated with medications. His current abdominal pain has localized to his right lower quadrant. He has had four CT scans over the last year, and recently had positive renal and bladder ultrasounds for urinary tract stones. What diagnostic imaging modality would be most beneficial?

Suggested Answer:
While the patient's history suggests multiple potential etiologies for his current symptoms, acute appendicitis is at the top of the differential. This study suggests that nonfocused abdominal and pelvic MDCT would be the best diagnostic imaging examination, and can assess for acute appendicitis as well as alternative diagnoses such as obstructive urinary tract stones and diverticulitis. The patient's recent imaging history should not dissuade you from approaching the acute diagnostic situation any differently than if the patient had had no recent diagnostic imaging.

References

1. Pickhardt PJ, Lawrence EM, Pooler BD, Bruce RJ. Diagnostic performance of multidetector computed tomography for suspected acute appendicitis. *Ann Intern Med.* 2011;154(12):789–796.
2. Rao PM, Rhea JT, Novelline RA, Mostafavi AA, McCabe CJ. Effect of computed tomography of the appendix on treatment of patients and use of hospital resources. *N Engl J Med.* 1998;338(3):141–146.
3. van Randen A, Bipat S, Zwinderman AH, Ubbink DT, Stoker J, Boermeester MA. Acute appendicitis: meta-analysis of diagnostic performance of CT and graded compression US related to prevalence of disease. *Radiology.* 2008;249(1):97–106.
4. Rosen MP, Ding A, Blake MA, et al. ACR Appropriateness Criteria right lower quadrant pain—suspected appendicitis. *J Am Coll Radiol.* 2011;8(11):749–755.

28

Uterine Artery Embolization for Fibroids

The Randomized Trial of Embolization versus Surgery Treatment for Fibroids (REST)

CHRISTOPH I. LEE

> In this randomized trial comparing uterine-artery embolization with standard surgical treatment for women with symptomatic fibroids, we found no significant differences between the groups in measures of quality of life at 12 months . . .
>
> —EDWARDS ET AL.[1]

Research Question: How effective is uterine artery embolization for treating symptomatic uterine fibroids versus surgery?

Funding: The Chief Scientific Office of the Scottish Executive, Edinburgh.

Year Study Began: 2000

Year Study Published: 2007

Study Location: 27 hospitals in the United Kingdom.

Who Was Studied: Women ≥18 years old, with symptomatic fibroid(s) >2 cm in size adequately visualized by MRI, who normally would undergo surgery (myomectomy or hysterectomy).

Who Was Excluded: Pregnant patients, patients unable to undergo MRI imaging, allergy to iodinated contrast, fibroid size <2 cm, subserosal pedunculated fibroids, recent or ongoing pelvic inflammatory disease, contraindication to surgery.

How Many Patients: 157

Study Overview: Randomized controlled trial. Randomization was stratified at the medical center level, with patients randomized in a 2:1 ratio, with twice as many patients allocated to the embolization group (n = 106) than the surgical group (n = 51; 43 hysterectomies, 8 myomectomies).

Study Intervention: Uterine artery embolizations were performed by experienced interventional radiologists and the study protocol required embolization of both uterine arteries with standardized particle size (500–710 μm) (Figures 28.1 and 28.2).

Follow-Up: Outcome measures assessed at 1, 6, 12, and 21 months and annually thereafter; 12-month follow-up results presented here.

Endpoints: Primary endpoint was quality of life, assessed at 12 months with the 36-item Short Form Health Survey (SF-36) quality of life questionnaire (scores ranging 0–100, higher scores indicating better function). Secondary endpoints were symptom scores, complications, return to lifestyle events, pain scores, and a cost minimization analysis.

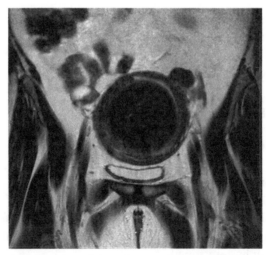

Figure 28.1 Coronal T1 image of the pelvis in a patient with a large uterine fibroid.

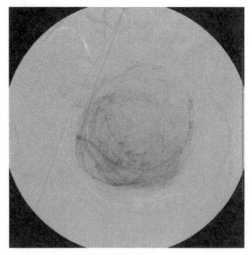

Figure 28.2 Digital subtraction angiography image as part of a uterine fibroid embolization procedure. Contrast was injected into a selected branch of the uterine artery, with visualization of the arteries supplying this patient's large uterine fibroid.

RESULTS

- After 1-year posttreatment, there were no statistically significant differences between groups in any of the eight components of the SF-36 scores (see Table 28.1).
- Patients in the embolization group had shorter median hospital stays (1 day vs. 5 days) and a shorter time to returning to work than the surgical group ($P < 0.001$ for both).
- While patients in the surgical group had higher pain scores at 24 hours, they had better symptom scores at 12 months ($P = 0.03$).
- There were similar rates of major adverse events during the first year of follow-up between groups: 12% (13/106) in embolization group, 20% (10/51) in surgical group ($P = 0.22$).
- After 1 year posttreatment, 13% (14/106) of women in the embolization group needed to be hospitalized, 3 with major adverse events and 11 for reintervention for treatment failure.
- A cost minimization analysis and one-way sensitivity analysis based on the trial's data suggested that, at 1 year, embolization was more cost-effective than surgery for patients with symptomatic uterine fibroids from a national payer perspective.

Table 28.1. THE TRIAL'S KEY FINDINGS

SF-36[a] Quality of Life Measure at 12 Months	Embolization Group	Surgical Group	P Value of Difference between Groups
Physical Function	92 ± 14	89 ± 20	0.85
Physical Role	76 ± 40	81 ± 34	0.33
Bodily Pain	76 ± 23	80 ± 26	0.28
General Health	74 ± 20	79 ± 17	0.07
Vitality	62 ± 21	67 ± 22	0.26
Social Function	84 ± 23	87 ± 26	0.35
Emotional Role	81 ± 35	87 ± 30	0.22
Mental Health	76 ± 17	76 ± 21	0.80

[a] SF-36 = Short-Form 36-item health survey.

Plus-minus values are means ± standard deviations. *P* value < 0.05 considered statistically significant.

Criticisms and Limitations: The SF-36 score does not take specific fibroid-related symptoms into account. Both hysterectomy and myomectomy patients were included, but only 8 women underwent myomectomy, making it difficult to compare the latter procedure to uterine artery embolization. The reported interval time to resumption of usual activities may have been biased by patients' expectations regarding time of recovery for differing procedure types.

Other Relevant Studies and Information:

- This trial's results support the finding of two previous randomized controlled trials that demonstrated significantly shorter hospital stays after uterine artery embolization compared to surgery.[2,3]
- A recent Cochrane Review of published trials, including longer-term follow-up data from the REST trial, found that there was no significant difference in reported quality of life two years following embolization versus surgery for symptomatic fibroids, and no clear evidence of a long-term difference between embolization and surgery for risk of major complications.[4]
- The American College of Radiology appropriateness criteria provide equal appropriateness ratings (7 out of 9) for uterine artery embolization and hysterectomy for women with symptomatic fibroids who no longer plan for future pregnancies.[5]

Summary and Implications: Women with symptomatic uterine fibroids undergoing uterine artery embolization have similar quality of life measures

1 year posttreatment and faster recovery after uterine artery embolization compared to surgery. However, benefits of noninvasive uterine artery embolization must be weighed against the need for reinterventions among a minority of patients with treatment failure.

CLINICAL CASE: UTERINE ARTERY EMBOLIZATION

Case History:
A 38-year-old female with menorrhagia and pelvic pain caused by a 7 cm uterine fibroid presents to your vascular and interventional clinic to discuss potential treatment options. She no longer desires future pregnancies and is concerned about the potential complications of surgery. What benefits and risks should you discuss regarding the option of uterine artery embolization?

Suggested Answer:
Based on the REST trial, the patient is equally likely to find quality-of-life benefits 1 year after treatment with either uterine artery embolization or hysterectomy. While there is little evidence to suggest more major adverse events from one procedure over the other, uterine artery embolization may lead to the need for reinterventions due to treatment failure among 13% of patients. Thus, while embolization may lead to quicker recovery given the relatively noninvasive technique, the higher potential treatment failure rate should be communicated to the patient as an associated risk.

References

1. Edwards RD, Moss JG, Lumsden MA, et al. Uterine-artery embolization versus surgery for symptomatic uterine fibroids. *N Engl J Med.* 2007;356(4):360–370.
2. Pinto I, Chimeno P, Romo A, et al. Uterine fibroids: uterine artery embolization versus abdominal hysterectomy for treatment—a prospective, randomized, and controlled clinical trial. *Radiology.* 2003;226:425–431.
3. Hehenkamp WJK, Volkers NA, Donderwinkel PFJ, et al. Uterine artery embolization versus hysterectomy in the treatment of symptomatic uterine fibroids (EMMY trial): peri- and postprocedural results from a randomized controlled trial. *Am J Obstet Gynecol.* 2005;193:1618–1629.
4. Gupta JK, Sinha A, Lumsden MA, Hickey M. Uterine artery embolization for symptomatic uterine fibroids. *Cochrane Database Syst Rev.* 2014;12:CD005073. doi:10.1002/14651858.CD005073.pub4.
5. Burke CT, Funaki BS, Ray CEJr, et al. ACR appropriateness criteria on treatment of uterine leiomyomas. *J Am Coll Radiol.* 2011;8(4):228–234.

29

Imaging for Suspected Nephrolithiasis

The Study of Tomography of Nephrolithiasis Evaluation (STONE) Trial

CHRISTOPH I. LEE

> ... using ultrasonography as the initial test in patients with suspected nephrolithiasis ... resulted in no need for CT in most patients, lower cumulative radiation exposure, and no significant differences in the risk of subsequent adverse events ...
>
> —Smith-Bindman et al.[1]

Research Question: Should the initial imaging examination for suspected nephrolithiasis be CT or ultrasound?

Funding: Agency for Healthcare Research and Quality.

Year Study Began: 2011

Year Study Published: 2014

Study Location: 15 large, urban, geographically diverse US emergency departments.

Who Was Studied: Men and women ages 18–75 years, presenting to the emergency department with flank or abdominal pain suggestive of acute renal colic.

Who Was Excluded: Children < 18 years; elderly patients ≥76 years; pregnant patients; morbidly obese patients (>285 lb if male, >250 lb if female); acute abdomen with signs of sepsis or alternative diagnosis; history of kidney problems (e.g., hemodialysis, kidney transplant, only one kidney).

How Many Patients: 2,759

Study Overview: Multicenter, randomized, pragmatic, comparative effectiveness trial.

Study Intervention: Patients were randomized to undergo imaging in a 1:1:1 ratio to 1 of 3 imaging groups: initial ultrasonography performed by an emergency physician (point-of-care ultrasonography, n = 908), initial ultrasonography performed by a radiologist (radiology ultrasonography, n = 893), or abdominal CT (n = 958). Management after initial imaging was at the discretion of treating physicians.

Follow-Up: Patient interviewed at 3, 7, 30, 90, and 180 days after randomization; review of medical records for resource utilization, radiation exposure, and diagnoses.

Endpoints: Primary endpoints were 30-day incidence of high-risk diagnoses that may represent complications related to missed or delayed diagnosis (e.g., abdominal aortic aneurysm rupture, pneumonia with sepsis, appendicitis with rupture, pyelonephritis with urosepsis) and 6-month cumulative radiation exposure (sum of effective doses for all imaging performed). Secondary endpoints were serious adverse events, pain (11-point visual-analogue score, higher scores indicating more severe pain), return emergency visits, hospitalizations, and diagnostic accuracy.

RESULTS

- Within the first 30 days, incidence of high-risk diagnoses with complications did not vary according to initial imaging method and were low across all groups ($P = 0.30$).
- The point-of-care ultrasonography and radiology ultrasonography groups had lower mean 6-month cumulative radiation exposure than the CT group ($P < 0.001$) (Table 29.1). This difference was attributable to baseline imaging during the emergency department visit.
- There was no significant difference in rate of serious adverse events (n = 466) across study groups ($P = 0.50$).
- The self-reported average pain score at 7 days, rate of return emergency visits (within 30 days), rate of hospitalization (within

Table 29.1. THE TRIAL'S KEY FINDINGS

Outcome	Point-of-Care Ultrasound (n = 908)	Radiology Ultrasound (n = 893)	Computed Tomography (n = 958)	P Value
High-risk diagnosis with complications— no. of patients (%)	6 (0.7)	3 (0.3)	2 (0.2)	0.30
Radiation exposure over 6 months— mean mSv (± SD)	10.1 ± 14.1	9.3 ± 13.4	17.2 ± 13.4	< 0.001
Serious adverse events—no. of patients (%)	113 (12.4)	96 (10.8)	107 (11.2)	0.50
Sensitivity for diagnosing nephrolithiasis— % (95% CI)	54 (48–60)	57 (51–64)	88 (84–92)	< 0.001
Specificity for diagnosing nephrolithiasis— % (95% CI)	71 (67–75)	73 (69–77)	58 (55–62)	< 0.001

mSv = millisieverts; SD = standard deviation; 95% CI = 95% confidence interval.
P value < 0.05 considered a statistically significant difference between groups.

180 days), and diagnostic accuracy (confirmed stone diagnosis within 6 months) did not differ significantly across groups.
- A CT scan was eventually performed in 41% of patients who initially underwent ultrasound; in contrast, only 5% of patients who initially underwent CT had a subsequent ultrasound.

Criticisms and Limitations: Investigators, patients, and physicians were not blinded to the initial imaging study group assignment. All emergency physicians were trained and certified in point-of-care ultrasound, which may not be true in many emergency department settings. While the prevalence of obesity is high among renal colic patients, obese patients were excluded from this study.

Other Relevant Studies and Information:

- Even though it imparts ionizing radiation, CT did have greater sensitivity for detecting nephrolithiasis compared to ultrasonography, but also had higher false-positive rates, findings that are consistent with prior studies.[2,3]

- Low-dose noncontrast CT can be performed at many medical centers, allowing identification of nephrolithiasis with similar diagnostic accuracy as standard CT with significantly reduced radiation dose.[4,5]
- For acute onset flank pain suspicious for stone disease, the American College of Radiology gives a higher appropriateness rating for CT abdomen and pelvis without contrast (reduced-dose techniques preferred, score 8 out of 9) than ultrasound of the kidneys and bladder (score 6 out of 9).[6]
- For recurrent symptoms of stone disease, the American College of Radiology gives the same appropriateness rating for CT abdomen and pelvis without contrast (reduced-dose techniques preferred) and ultrasound of the kidneys and bladder (score 7 out of 9 for both).[6]

Summary and Implications: Initial imaging with ultrasonography for suspected nephrolithiasis has similar diagnostic accuracy and short-term patient outcomes (e.g., high-risk diagnoses with complications, serious adverse events, pain scores, hospitalizations) but is associated with lower cumulative radiation exposure, compared to initial imaging with CT for suspected nephrolithiasis. Thus, ultrasound should be used as the initial diagnostic imaging test for patients with suspected renal colic, with additional imaging performed (e.g., CT) as needed (Figure 29.1).

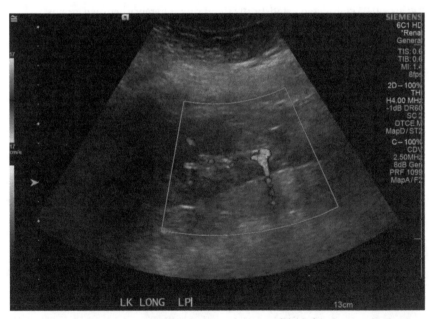

Figure 29.1 Sagittal color Doppler ultrasound image of the left kidney with a large lower-pole renal calculus. Note the "twinkle" artifact extending posteriorly from the calculus. This is a classic finding when applying color Doppler to a renal calculus.

CLINICAL CASE: INITIAL IMAGING FOR RENAL COLIC

Case History:

A 56-year-old male presents with sudden, severe left flank pain that seems to get worse in waves. He complains of nausea and vomiting for several hours, and his laboratory results demonstrate hematuria. What imaging study should you perform first?

Suggested Answer:

Results from the STONE trial suggest that ultrasound of the kidneys and bladder should be considered as the first-line imaging modality, with CT a consideration if the ultrasound is inconclusive or the symptoms continue to be highly suggestive of renal colic. A significant proportion of patients in the STONE trial undergoing ultrasound first eventually did obtain a CT scan. If CT is needed, a low-dose protocol and no intravenous contrast are preferred.

References

1. Smith-Bindman R, Aubin C, Bailitz J, et al. Ultrasonography versus computed tomography for suspected nephrolithiasis. *N Engl J Med.* 2014;371(12):1100–1110.
2. Worster A, Preyra I, Weaver B, Haines T. The accuracy of noncontrast helical computed tomography versus intravenous pyelography in the diagnosis of suspected acute urolithiasis: a meta-analysis. *Ann Emerg Med.* 2002;40(3):280–286.
3. Edmonds ML, Yan JW, Sedran RJ, McLeod SL, Theakston KD. The utility of renal ultrasonography in the diagnosis of renal colic in emergency department patients. *Can J Emer Med.* 2010;12(3):201–206.
4. Zilberman DE, Tsivian M, Lipkin ME, et al. Low dose computerized tomography for detection of urolithiasis—its effectiveness in the setting of the urology clinic. *J Urol.* 2011;185(3):910–914.
5. Jellison FC, Smith JC, Heldt JP, et al. Effect of low dose radiation computerized tomography protocols on distal ureteral calculus detection. *J Urol.* 2009;182(6):2762–2767.
6. Coursey CA, Casalino DD, Remer EM, et al. ACR Appropriateness Criteria® acute onset flank pain—suspicion of stone disease. *Ultrasound Q.* 2012;28(3):227–233.

30

Imaging-Guided Biopsy for Diagnosing Prostate Cancer

CHIRSTOPH I. LEE

> The number needed to biopsy by standard biopsy in addition to targeted [MR/ultrasound fusion] biopsy to diagnose 1 additional high-risk tumor was 200 men.
>
> —SIDDIQUI ET AL.[1]

Research Question: What type of imaging-guided biopsy is more accurate for diagnosing high-risk prostate cancer?

Funding: National Institutes of Health (Intramural Research Program of the NIH, National Cancer Institute, Center for Cancer Research, and Center for Interventional Oncology).

Year Study Began: 2007

Year Study Published: 2015

Study Location: National Cancer Institute in Bethesda, MD.

Who Was Studied: Men referred with elevated prostate-specific antigen (PSA) or abnormal digital rectal examination and multiparametric prostate MRI demonstrating at least one lesion in the prostate.

Who Was Excluded: Men with prior prostate cancer therapy and contraindication for multiparametric MRI.

How Many Patients: 1,003

Study Overview: Prospective clinical trial of men suspected of having prostate
cancer that underwent multiparametric MRI. The MRI studies were evaluated
in a blinded format with lesions assigned low, moderate, or high suspicion scores
by two highly experienced genitourinary radiologists (8 and 14 years of experience interpreting prostate multiparametric MRI). Patients with suspicious
MRI findings underwent concurrent targeted MR/ultrasound fusion prostate
biopsy (biopsy system superimposing previously identified MRI lesion on to
real-time transrectal ultrasound images) and standard extended-sextant biopsy
(12 core biopsies using a template covering the lateral and medial aspects of
the base, mid, and apical prostate). More biopsy cores were obtained as part of
standard biopsy if an ultrasound abnormality was noted.

Study Intervention: Patients underwent multiparametric prostate MRI on a
3.0-tesla MRI with four sequences: triplanar T2-weighted, dynamic contrast-
enhanced, diffusion-weighted imaging, and MR spectroscopy (Figure 30.1).
Imaging was followed by targeted MR/ultrasound fusion biopsy and standard
biopsy, concurrently.

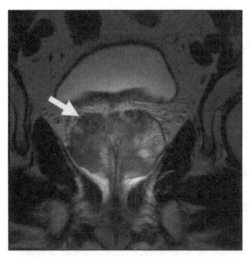

Figure 30.1 Coronal T2 MRI image of the prostate demonstrating a small focus of
hypointensity within the right peripheral zone of the prostate, representing prostate
carcinoma (arrow). Image courtesy of Veronica Cox, MD; MD Anderson Cancer Center.

Follow-Up: None reported.

Endpoints: Primary endpoint was detection of high-risk prostate cancer (Gleason score $\geq 4 + 3$). Secondary endpoints were detection of low-risk prostate cancer (Gleason score $3 + 3$ or low-volume $3 + 4$) and ability to predict whole-gland pathology at prostatectomy (the gold standard when available).

RESULTS

- Targeted MR/ultrasound fusion biopsy diagnosed 30% more high-risk prostate cancers (173 vs. 122 cases, $P < 0.001$) and 17% fewer low-risk prostate cancers (213 vs. 258 cases, $P < 0.001$) (Table 30.1).
- Adding standard biopsy to the targeted approach yielded an additional 103 (22%) cases of prostate cancers, mostly low-risk cancers (83% low risk, 12% intermediate risk, and 5% high risk).
- Adding standard biopsy to targeted biopsy did not change Gleason score risk stratification in 85% of cases (857/1003). Of those with a risk stratification change, only 2% (19/1,003) increased to high-risk prostate cancer.
- Among 170 men with whole-gland pathology after prostatectomy, targeted fusion biopsy had higher predictive ability for differentiating low-risk from intermediate- and high-risk disease compared to standard biopsy or the two approaches combined (area under the curve, 0.73, 0.59, and 0.67, respectively, $P < 0.05$) (Table 30.2).

Table 30.1. COMPARISON OF PATIENTS' PATHOLOGY BASED ON BIOPSY TECHNIQUE

Targeted MR/ Ultrasound Fusion Biopsy	Standard Extended-Sextant Biopsy			
	No Cancer	Low-Risk Cancer[a]	Intermediate-Risk Cancer[b]	High-Risk Cancer[c]
No Cancer	439	86	12	5
Low-Risk Cancer[a]	55	119	29	10
Intermediate-Risk Cancer[b]	14	28	29	4
High-Risk Cancer[c]	26	25	19	103

[a] Low-risk cancer: Gleason 6 or Gleason $3 + 4$ low volume.
[b] Intermediate-risk cancer: Gleason $3 + 4$ high volume.
[c] High-risk cancer: Gleason $\geq 4 + 3$.

Table 30.2. BIOPSY APPROACH PERFORMANCE FOR DETECTING
INTERMEDIATE- OR HIGH-RISK PROSTATE CANCER

Performance Characteristic % (95% CI)	Targeted MR/ Ultrasound Fusion Biopsy	Standard Extended-Sextant Biopsy	Combined Biopsy
Sensitivity	77 (67–84)	53 (43–63)	85 (76–91)
Specificity	68 (57–78)	66 (54–76)	49 (37–60)
Negative predictive value	70 (58–80)	53 (43–63)	73 (58–84)
Positive predictive value	75 (65–83)	66 (54–76)	67 (58–75)
Area under the curve	0.73 (0.66–0.79)	0.59 (0.52–0.67)	0.67 (0.60–0.74)

Criticisms and Limitations: The majority of patients had at least one previous prostate biopsy, suggesting selection bias. Assigned suspicion scores for MRI findings did not utilize standardized Prostate Imaging Reporting and Data System (PI-RADS) criteria. Highly experienced genitourinary radiologists interpreted all MRI studies, and accuracy may be worse in other settings without experienced readers. The study is preliminary with regards to clinical endpoints including disease recurrence and prostate cancer–specific mortality. Fusion MR/ultrasound biopsy is more expensive and not widely accessible.

Other Relevant Studies and Information:

- Traditionally, prostate cancer has been diagnosed with random sampling of the entire organ using a standard extended-sextant biopsy technique. The recent introduction of multiparametric MRI has allowed for image-based identification of focal areas of prostate cancer,[2] and fusion with transrectal ultrasound images has made targeted biopsy of suspicious regions possible.[3]
- Early clinical trials of combined targeted biopsy and standard biopsy suggest that combined biopsy is more accurate than standard biopsy alone for detecting clinically significant prostate cancers.[4]
- A systematic review of MR-targeted prostate biopsy concluded that fusion biopsy can detect clinically significant cancers with fewer core samples compared with usual sampling techniques, and that the use of MR may eliminate the need for biopsy in one-third of men and may avoid a diagnosis of clinically insignificant cancer.[5]

- The National Comprehensive Care Network and the American Urological Association recommend an extended-pattern 12-core biopsy that includes the standard sextant approach for initial prostate transrectal ultrasound-guided biopsy.[6]

Summary and Implications: Targeted MR/ultrasound fusion biopsy among men with suspected prostate cancer, compared to standard extended-sextant ultrasound-guided biopsy, is associated with higher detection of high-risk prostate cancer and lower detection of low-risk prostate cancer. In addition, targeted biopsy may significantly shift the distribution of risk in men newly diagnosed with prostate cancer toward more high-risk disease.

CLINICAL CASE: IMAGING-GUIDED PROSTATE BIOPSY

Case History:
A 58-year-old male presents to your primary care clinic to discuss his prostate cancer screening results. His PSA level was high at 8 ng/mL. He would like to discuss the risks and benefits of further workup and expresses his desire to undergo biopsy. He is particularly interested in a newer method for biopsy he has been reading about online—the MR/ultrasound fusion-guided biopsy. How would you advise this patient?

Suggested Answer:
Most experts agree that a total PSA of 4.0 ng/mL or higher is the threshold for being considered abnormal and requiring referral for biopsy.[6] The standard of care is extended sextant-biopsy with transrectal ultrasound guidance. With regard to MR/ultrasound fusion guided biopsy, you should inform your patient that, while preliminary reports are promising, there are no randomized clinical trials examining whether this new diagnostic technique leads to improved clinical outcomes. However, the patient is in-network with the academic medical center offering this service. If the patient has no contraindications to MRI, he could choose this diagnostic option, with the caveat of potential increased out-of-pocket costs.

References

1. Siddiqui MM, Rais-Bahrami S, Turkbey B, et al. Comparison of MR/ultrasound fusion-guided biopsy with ultrasound-guided biopsy for the diagnosis of prostate cancer. *JAMA*. 2015;313(4):390–397.

2. Fütterer JJ, Heijmink SW, Scheenen TW, et al. Prostate cancer localization with dynamic contrast-enhanced MR imaging and proton MR spectroscopic imaging. *Radiology.* 2006;241(2):449–458.

3. Siddiqui MM, Rais-Bahrami S, Truong H, et al. Magnetic resonance imaging/ultrasound-fusion biopsy significantly upgrades prostate cancer versus systematic 12-core transrectal ultrasound biopsy. *Eur Urol.* 2013;64(5):713–719.

4. Wysock JS, Rosenkrantz AB, Huang WC, et al. A prospective, blinded comparison of magnetic resonance (MR) imaging-ultrasound fusion and visual estimation in the performance of MR-targeted prostate biopsy: the PROFUS trial. *Eur Urol.* 2014;66(2):343–351.

5. Moore CM, Robertson NL, Arsanious N, et al. Image-guided prostate biopsy using magnetic resonance imaging-derived targets: a systematic review. *Eur Urol.* 2013;63(1):125–140.

6. Gulati R, Gore JL, Etzioni R. Comparative effectiveness of alternative prostate-specific antigen-based prostate cancer screening strategies: model estimates of potential benefits and harms. *Ann Intern Med.* 2013;158(3):145–153.

Bone, Joint, and Extremity Pain

31

Decision Rules for Imaging Acute Ankle Injuries

The Ottawa Ankle Rules

CHRISTOPH I. LEE

> Application of the decision rules . . . would have led to relative reductions in the proportion of patients referred for ankle series radiography by 34% . . . and for foot series radiography by 30% . . .
>
> —STIELL ET AL.[1]

Research Question: Can a decision rule allow physicians to safely forego x-rays in patients with acute ankle injuries?

Funding: None reported.

Year Study Began: 1991

Year Study Published: 1993

Study Location: Two Canadian university-affiliated emergency departments.

Who Was Studied: Adults with blunt, acute ankle trauma.

Who Was Excluded: Patients <18 years, who are pregnant, have isolated injuries to the skin, were referred from outside hospital with radiography, with ankle injury >10 days previous, and are returning for reassessment of same injury.

How Many Patients: 1,032 in the first stage and 453 in the second stage

Study Overview: Refinement of previously derived decision rules (first stage) followed by validation of refined rules (second stage). Attending emergency physicians assessed each patient presenting with acute ankle trauma for standardized variables and classified the need for radiography. Interobserver reliability was examined by having a second emergency physician assess the same patients in a blinded fashion when feasible. Original decision rules were refined using univariate and recursive partitioning analyses toward the objective of 100% sensitivity for fractures with maximum possible specificity. These refined criteria were validated in a separate set of patients presenting with acute ankle injury.

Study Intervention: Staff emergency physicians evaluated each participant for standardized clinical variables. All patients underwent radiography, including a standard ankle series if pain is in the malleolar region, or standard foot series if pain is in the midfoot zone. Staff radiologists interpreted all images blinded to the content of the data collection forms.

Follow-Up: None.

Endpoints: Clinically significant fractures of the malleoli and midfoot (defined as bone fragments >3 mm in breadth) (Figure 31.1).

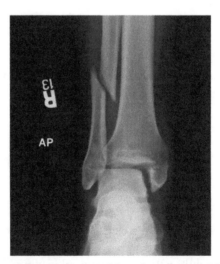

Figure 31.1 AP radiograph of the right ankle with complex ankle fracture involving the distal fibular diaphysis and medial malleolus. Soft tissue injury is also likely given displacement of the fracture fragments and subluxation of the distal tibia on the talus.

RESULTS

- The original decision rule had 100% sensitivity (95% CI, 97%–100%) for detecting 121 malleolar zone factures and 98% (95% CI, 88%–100%) for detecting 49 midfoot zone fractures.
- The refined decision rule after recursive partitioning had 100% sensitivity (95% CI, 93%–100%) for 50 malleolar zone fractures and 100% (95% CI, 83%–100%) for 19 midfoot zone fractures (Box 31.1).
- The refined decision rule achieved a slightly higher specificity than the original rule (41% vs. 39%).
- The probability of fracture given a negative decision rule is estimated as 0% (95% CI, 0%–0.8%) in ankle series and 0% (95% CI, 0%–0.4%) in foot series.

Box 31.1. THE OTTAWA ANKLE RULE

Ankle x-ray is only required if there is malleolar zone pain and any of the below:

- Bone tenderness along distal 6 cm of posterior edge of tibia or tip of medial malleolus.
- Bone tenderness along distal 6 cm of posterior edge of fibula or tip of lateral malleolus.
- Inability to bear weight both immediately and in emergency department for four steps.

Foot x-ray is only required if there is midfoot zone pain and any of the below:

- Bone tenderness at base of the fifth metatarsal.
- Bone tenderness at navicular bone.
- Inability to bear weight both immediately and in emergency department for four steps.

Criticisms and Limitations: This was a convenience sample of adult patients at two university-affiliated hospitals in Canada. The Ottawa Ankle Rules were developed and validated for adult patients, so they may not reliably be extended to the pediatric population.

Other Relevant Studies and Information:

- One systematic review pooled data from 27 studies regarding ankle and foot injury assessment, and found a baseline prevalence of 15% acute fractures in patient presenting with ankle or foot trauma and a probability of fracture after negative Ottawa rule assessment of <1.4%.[2]
- This same systematic review found a pooled sensitivity of 97.6% for the Ottawa Ankle Rules and a median specificity of 31.5%.[2]
- In children (≤16 years), the Ottawa Ankle Rules also have a high sensitivity (1.0, 95% CI .95–1.0) for malleolar fractures and midfoot fractures (1.0, 95% CI, 0.82–1.0).[3]
- The Buffalo rule is similar to the Ottawa Ankle Rules but directs point tenderness criterion to the crest or midportion of the malleoli (distal 6 cm of the fibular and tibia), which is meant to decrease likelihood of palpating over ligament structures. The Buffalo rule had 100% sensitivity (95% CI, 59%–100%) and 59% specificity (95% CI, 47%–71%) for fracture in the setting of malleolar pain.[4]
- ACR Appropriateness Criteria abide by the Ottawa Ankle Rules, and rate an ankle radiograph series as highly appropriate (score 9 out of 9) when a patient meets the Ottawa Ankle Rules criteria.[5]
- Ankle MRI may be an important secondary examination when tendon or ligament tears, or osteochondral and cartilage abnormalities, are suspected.[6]

Summary and Implications: The refined and validated Ottawa Ankle Rules have the potential to reduce approximately 30%–34% of all foot and ankle radiographs for acute injuries, with 100% sensitivity for reliably detecting foot and ankle fractures.

CLINICAL CASE: ACUTE ANKLE INJURY

Case History:
A 32-year-old male presents to the emergency room after a bicycle accident complaining of acute right ankle pain, centered about the malleolar zone. He was unable to bear weight immediately but is able to take several steps in the emergency department with some pain. On physical exam, there is no focal bone tenderness along the majority of the distal tibia and fibula, or at the lateral malleolus. There is only focal bone tenderness at the medial malleolus. Should you order an ankle radiograph series to rule out an acute fracture?

Suggested Answer:
According to the Ottawa Ankle Rules, focal bone pain only at the medial malleolus should push you toward ordering an ankle radiograph series. Even without other areas of focal pain and improved ability to bear weight, focal bone pain at the medial malleolus alone is enough to require radiographic examination to rule out an acute ankle fracture.

References

1. Stiell IG, Greenberg GH, McKnight RD, et al. Decision rules for the use of radiography in acute ankle injuries. Refinement and prospective validation. *JAMA*. 1993;269(9):1127–1132.
2. Bachmann LM, Kolb E, Koller MT, et al. Accuracy of Ottawa ankle rules to exclude fractures of the ankle and mid-foot: systematic review. *BMJ*. 2003;326(7386):417–423.
3. Plint AC, Bulloch B, Osmond MH, et al. Validation of the Ottawa Ankle Rules in children with ankle injuries. *Acad Emerg Med*. 1999;6(10):1005–1009.
4. Leddy JJ, Smolinksi RJ, Lawrence J, Snyder JL, Priore RL. Prospective evaluation of the Ottawa Ankle Rules in a university sports medicine center: with a modification to increase specificity for identifying malleolar fractures. *Am J Sports Med*. 1998;26(2):158–165.
5. American College of Radiology. ACR Appropriateness Criteria for acute trauma to the ankle. https://acsearch.acr.org/docs/69436/Narrative/. Published 1995. Updated 2014. Accessed December 6, 2015.
6. Papaliodis DN, Vanushkina MA, Richardson NG, DiPreta JA. The foot and ankle examination. *Med Clin North Am*. 2014;98(2):181–204.

32

Decision Rule for Imaging Acute Knee Injuries

The Ottawa Knee Rules

CHRISTOPH I. LEE

> Physicians can be confident that if radiography is ordered according to the decision rule the likelihood of missing a clinically important fracture is remote.
>
> —STIELL ET AL.[1]

Research Question: Can a decision rule allow physicians to safely forego x-rays in patients with acute knee injuries?

Funding: None reported.

Year Study Began: 1994.

Year Study Published: 1996.

Study Location: Two Canadian, university-affiliated emergency departments.

Who Was Studied: Adults with blunt acute knee trauma, broadly defined to include the patella, head and neck of the fibula, proximal 8 cm of the tibia, and distal 8 cm of the femur.

Who Was Excluded: Patients <18 years, pregnant patients, patients referred from an outside hospital with knee radiographs, patients with isolated injuries of the skin, knee injury >7 days previous, patients returning for reassessment of same injury, altered level of consciousness, paraplegic, or patients with multiple injuries.

How Many Patients: 1,096

Study Overview: Emergency physicians prospectively assessed each patient for 14 standardized clinical variables and determined the need for imaging based on the decision rule. The rule was assessed for ability to identify knee fractures and was then refined by univariate and recursive partitioning analyses.

Study Intervention: Knee radiography series were ordered according to usual care practices of individual physicians. Radiographs were interpreted by radiologists blinded to the data collection sheet contents.

Follow-Up: Structured telephone interview at day 14 for patients who did not undergo radiography to assess possibility of fracture among patients discharged without radiography.

Endpoints: Clinically important fracture demonstrated on a standard knee radiography series as determined by a consensus of orthopedic surgeons and emergency physicians at the University of Ottawa. These were defined as any bone fragment at least 5 mm in breadth or any avulsion fracture if associated with complete disruption of tendons or ligaments (Figure 32.1).

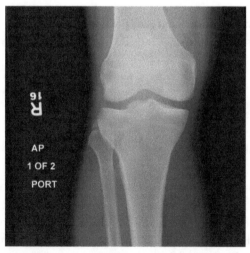

Figure 32.1 AP radiograph of the right knee with inferiorly displaced fracture of the lateral tibial plateau. Note the associated mildly displaced fracture of the fibular head.

RESULTS

- The decision rule had 100% sensitivity (95% CI, 94%–100%) for identifying 63 clinically significant fractures (63/1096, 6% of patients) (Box 32.1).
- Among 357 patients discharged without radiography, none required reassessment after the follow-up telephone interview.
- Emergency physicians correctly interpreted the rule 96% of the time, and would not have missed any fractures due to misinterpretation.
- Physician interobserver agreement was excellent, with a kappa value of 0.77 (95% CI, 0.65–0.89).
- Utilization of the decision rule would have led to a relative reduction in knee radiography of 28% (from 74% baseline to 53%).

Box 32.1. THE DECISION RULE FOR RADIOGRAPHY IN ACUTE KNEE INJURIES

Knee x-ray series is only required in acute knee injury patients with at least one of the following:

- Age ≥ 55 years
- Tenderness at head of fibula
- Isolated tenderness of patella
- Inability to flex to 90 degrees
- Inability to bear weight both immediately and in the emergency department for four steps

---

Criticisms and Limitations: Not all patients underwent knee radiography; however, a structured telephone interview at 2-week follow-up was used to mitigate the possibility of missed fractures. The decision rule was not tested in patients <18 years old.

Other Relevant Studies and Information:

- The Pittsburgh decision rule suggests knee radiograph series in blunt trauma or a fall as mechanism of injury plus either of the following: (1) age <12 years or >50 years, or (2) inability to walk 4 weight-bearing steps at the time of evaluation.[2]
- A prospective study comparing the Ottawa and Pittsburgh decision rules in three teaching hospitals showed that the Pittsburgh decision

rules were 99% sensitive and 60% specific for knee fractures, while the Ottawa knee rules were 97% sensitive and 27% specific for knee fractures.[3]

- ACR Appropriateness Criteria rate a knee radiograph series as a highly appropriate (score 9 out of 9) first-line study in the setting of acute knee injury with focal tenderness, effusion, or inability to bear weight.[4]
- Knee MRI may be an important secondary exam in cases with suspected meniscal tears, ligamentous tears, articular cartilage infractions, and extensor mechanism abnormalities.[5]

Summary and Implications: The Ottawa Knee Rule is highly accurate, reliable, and acceptable to emergency physicians. Adherence to the decision rule has the potential to reduce unnecessary radiography in acute knee injury cases by 28%.

CLINICAL CASE: ACUTE KNEE INJURY

Case History:
A 22-year-old female presents to the emergency room after sliding on her knees during a soccer match. The patient complains of focal right knee pain. On physical examination, she has soft tissue abrasions over her right knee, is able to flex her right knee to 90 degrees, can bear weight for several steps, and has no tenderness at the head of the fibula. The only positive sign on physical examination is focal tenderness over the right patella. Should you order a standard knee radiograph series?

Suggested Answer:
Based on the Ottawa knee rule, isolated focal tenderness over the patella is an indication for ordering a standard radiograph series. Isolated tenderness over the patella is an important clinical finding, as not intervening on a significant patellar fracture could lead to loss of the full extensor mechanism and mobility of the knee. Early intervention of patellar fractures can have significant affects on eventual outcomes.

References

1. Stiell IG, Greenberg GH, Wells GA, et al. Prospective validation of a decision rule for the use of radiography in acute knee injuries. *JAMA.* 1996; 275(8):611–615.

2. Bauer SJ, Hollander JE, Fuchs SH, Thode HCJr. A clinical decision rule in the evaluation of acute knee injuries. *J Emerg Med.* 1995;13(5):611–615.

3. Seaberg DC, Yealy DM, Lukens T, Auble T, Mathias S. Multicenter comparison of two clinical decision rules for the use of radiography in acute, high-risk knee injuries. *Ann Emerg Med.* 1998;32(1):8–13.

4. American College of Radiology. ACR Appropriateness Criteria for acute trauma to the knee. https://acsearch.acr.org/docs/69419/Narrative/. Published 1998. Revised 2014. Accessed December 4, 2015.

5. Oei EH, Ginai AZ, Hunink MG. MRI for traumatic knee injury: a review. *Semin Ultrasound CT MR.* 2007;28(2):141–157.

33

Incidental Meniscal Findings on Knee MRI

CHRISTOPH I. LEE

Clinicians who order MRI of the knee should take into account the high prevalence of incidental tears when interpreting the results and planning therapy.

—ENGLUND ET AL.[1]

Research Question: Are incidental meniscal tears seen on knee MRI clinically significant and associated with knee symptoms?

Funding: National Institutes of Health, Swedish Research Council, the Tegger Foundation, and the Arthritis Foundation.

Year Study Began: 2002

Year Study Published: 2008

Study Location: Single academic medical center.

Who Was Studied: Adults at least 50 years of age from Framingham, Massachusetts, drawn from 2000 census-tract data and random-digit telephone dialing. Adults needed to be ambulatory (assistive devices, such as canes, allowed).

Who Was Excluded: Subjects with a history of bilateral total knee replacement, rheumatoid arthritis, dementia, terminal cancer, or contraindication to MRI.

How Many Patients: 991

Study Overview: MRI scans of the knee were obtained on all study participants using a standardized imaging protocol (three pulse sequences: sagittal
and coronal fat-saturated, proton-density-weighted, turbo spin-echo images).
Scans were read by an orthopedist with confirmation by a musculoskeletal
radiologist. Interobserver agreement for MRI detection of meniscal damage
was excellent ($\kappa = 0.72$). One musculoskeletal radiologist, unaware of MRI
findings, graded weight-bearing posteroanterior knee radiographs with fixed-
flexion protocol according to the Kellgren-Lawrence scale.[2] Participants completed a questionnaire concerning knee joint symptoms.

Study Interventions: 1.5-tesla MRI with a phased-array knee coil was used to
assess for integrity of the menisci in the right knee. Weight-bearing posteroanterior knee radiographs with use of a fixed-flexion protocol and written questionnaire evaluating knee symptoms were also used.

Follow-Up: None reported.

Endpoints: On MRI, increased meniscal signal was deemed indicative of
meniscal tear when it communicated with inferior, superior, or free edge of
meniscal surface on at least two consecutive images (Figure 33.1). Absence
of meniscal tissue was deemed indicative of meniscal destruction. On radiographs, tibiofemoral osteoarthritis was considered present if Kellgren-
Lawrence grade was ≥2 (on scale 0–4, with higher numbers indicative of more

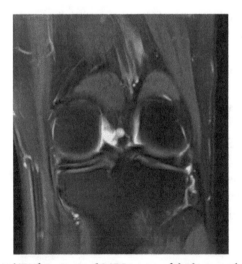

Figure 33.1 Coronal T2 fat-saturated MRI image of the knee with a horizontal tear
of the medial meniscus.

definitive osteoarthritis). The primary study endpoint was prevalence of meniscal findings on MRI, with a 95% confidence interval.

RESULTS

- Overall, the prevalence of meniscal damage in the right knee was 35% (95% CI, 32%–38%). Prevalence of meniscal tear was 31% (95% CI, 28%–34%) and prevalence of meniscal destruction was 10% (95% CI, 8%–12%) (Table 33.1).
- Prevalence of meniscal damage increased with age ($P < 0.001$ for trend). Prevalence was 32% (95% CI, 26%–40%) in men and 19% (95% CI, 15%–24%) in women 50–59 years old, compared to 56% (95% CI, 46%–66%) in men and 51% (95% CI, 42%–60%) among women 70–90 years old.
- Prevalence of meniscal damage was significantly higher among those with evidence of tibiofemoral osteoarthritis with increasing prevalence by severity (higher Kellgren-Lawrence grade, $P < 0.001$ for trend).
- No statistically significant differences in proportion of persons who had pain or stiffness symptoms according to type of tear, compartment of tear, or extension of tear into the peripheral third off the meniscus.

Table 33.1. THE TRIAL'S KEY FINDINGS

Meniscal Tears	Frequent Knee Symptoms No. (%)		Prevalence Ratio[a] Value (95% CI)
	Yes	No	
Imaging evidence of osteoarthritis			
Meniscal tear(s)	57 (63%)	46 (60%)	1.14 (0.90–1.45)
No meniscal tear	33 (37%)	31 (40%)	
No imaging evidence of osteoarthritis			1.43 (1.08–1.90)
Meniscal tear(s)	41 (32%)	146 (23%)	
No meniscal tear	86 (68%)	502 (77%)	

[a] Prevalence ratio (adjusted for age, sex, and body mass index) calculated as proportion of participants with meniscal tears among those with frequent knee symptoms divided by corresponding proportion without frequent knee symptoms.

Criticisms and Limitations: Recruitment by random-digit dialing may have led to some selection bias, affecting the prevalence estimates. The population was primarily Caucasian and residing in a suburban setting, which may limit generalizability to other sociodemographic groups. Study results are not generalizable to younger populations, whose meniscal tears may be more likely to correspond with symptoms. The study did not differentiate or identify types of meniscal tears that may been unstable and at increased risk of mechanical symptoms.

Other Relevant Studies and Information:

- Meniscal tears in the knee are the most frequent orthopedic diagnosis leading to arthroscopic partial meniscectomy, one of the most frequent orthopedic surgeries performed in the United States. Those undergoing this procedure are at increased risk for subsequent osteoarthritis.[3]
- Previous studies have reported a high prevalence of meniscal damage (67%–91%) among individuals with symptomatic knee osteoarthritis.[4,5]
- MRI is accurate in detecting meniscal tear, with sensitivity ranging between 79%–93% and specificity ranging between 88%–95%.[6]

Summary and Implications: Incidental meniscal damage on MRI is common in the general population, especially among the elderly, and is not necessarily attributable to patients' knee symptoms. Those interpreting MRI reports and planning interventions should realize that there is a high prevalence of incidental tears even among those without knee symptoms.

CLINICAL CASE: MENISCAL TEAR ON KNEE MRI

Case History:
A 56-year-old male with chronic knee pain under your care has just undergone a knee MRI. The radiology report indicates moderate tibiofemoral osteoarthritis and some signal abnormality in posterior horn of the medial meniscus, suggestive of a meniscal tear. Otherwise, there is no evidence of other structure damage or derangement. Should you refer your patient to an orthopedic surgeon for arthroscopic partial meniscectomy?

Suggested Answer:
In this study, among the 308 persons with a meniscal tear in their right knee, 66% had a medial tear. Among those with a tear, 66% had a tear involving the posterior horn of the meniscus. Thus, this case represents the most common incidental finding on knee MRI. Since there is baseline high prevalence of meniscal damage in the general population, you should advise your patient that this is a common finding that may or may not be associated with his chronic knee pain. Before referring the patient to an orthopedic surgeon, you should counsel the patient about the risks and benefits of interventions for nonspecific symptoms such as generalized knee pain.[7]

References

1. Englund M, Guermazi A, Gale D, et al. Incidental meniscal findings on knee MRI in middle-aged and elderly persons. *N Engl J Med*. 2008;359(11):1108–1115.
2. Felson DT, Naimark A, Anderson J, Kazis L, Castelli W, Meenan RF. The prevalence of knee osteoarthritis in the elderly: the Framingham Osteoarthritis Study. *Arthritis Rheum*. 1987;30(8):914–918.
3. Englund M, Lohmander LS. Risk factors for symptomatic knee osteoarthritis fifteen to twenty-two years after meniscectomy. *Arthritis Rheum*. 2004;50(9):2811–2819.
4. Englund M, Niu J, Guermazi A, et al. Effect of meniscal damage on the development of frequent knee pain, aching, or stiffness. *Arthritis Rheum*. 2007;56(12):4048–4054.
5. Kornaat PR, Bloem JL, Ceulemans RY, et al. Osteoarthritis of the knee: association between clinical features and MR imaging findings. *Radiology* 2006; 239(3):811–817.
6. Fox MG. MR imaging of the meniscus: review, current trends, and clinical implications. *Radiol Clin North Am*. 2007;45(6):1033–1053.
7. Sihvonen R, Paavola M, Malmivaara A, et al. Arthroscopic partial meniscectomy versus sham surgery for a degenerative meniscal tear. *N Engl J Med*. 2013;369(26):2515–2524.

34

Decision Rules for Bone Densitometry Testing

CHRISTOPH I. LEE

The SCORE [Simple Calculated Osteoporosis Risk Estimation] and ORAI [Osteoporosis Risk Assessment Instrument] decision rules are better than NOF [National Osteoporosis Foundation] guidelines at targeting BMD [bone mineral density] testing in high-risk patients.

—CADARETTE ET AL.[1]

Research Question: Which decision rule performs the best at selecting women for dual-energy x-ray absorptiometry (DEXA) screening for osteoporosis?

Funding: National Health Research and Development Program, Medical Research Council of Canada, MRC-PMAC Health Program, Merck Frosst Canada, Eli Lilly Canada, Procter & Gamble Canada, and the Dairy Farmers of Canada.

Year Study Began: 1996

Year Study Published: 2001

Study Location: Six study centers across Canada, located in Calgary, Halifax, Québec City, Saskatoon, St. John's, and Vancouver.

Who Was Studied: Postmenopausal women ≥45 years of age. The study sample was from the baseline data collection of a population-based, 5-year cohort study called the Canadian Multicentre Osteoporosis Study (CaMos), which evaluated the relationship between risk factors for osteoporosis, measures of bone mineral density, and osteoporotic fracture.

Who Was Excluded: Women with physician-diagnosed bone disease, at high risk for secondary osteoporosis, taking bone-sparing medication other than ovarian hormones, taking hormone replacement therapy for <5 years, or missing data for any risk factor required for decision rules.

How Many Patients: 2,365

Table 34.1. PATIENT SELECTION CRITERIA FOR BONE MINERAL
DENSITY TESTING

Rule/Guideline	Selection Threshold	Scoring(Points)
ABONE (Age, Body Size, No Estrogen)	Score ≥ 2	Age: > 65 years (1) Weight: < 63.5 kg (1) Estrogen use: Never used oral contraceptives or estrogen therapy ≥ 6 months (1)
NOF (National Osteoporosis Foundation)	Score ≥ 1	Age: ≥ 65 years (1) Weight: < 57.6 kg (1) Personal minimum trauma fracture ≥ 40 years (1) Family history of fracture (1) Current smoker (1)
ORAI (Osteoporosis Risk Assessment Instrument)	Score ≥ 9	Age: ≥ 75 years (15), 65–74 years (9), 55–64 years (5) Weight: < 60 kg (9), 60–69.9 kg (3) Estrogen use: Not currently taking estrogen (2)
SCORE (Simple Calculated Osteoporosis Risk Estimation)	Score ≥ 6	Race: Not black (5) Rheumatoid arthritis (4) Personal minimal trauma fracture after age 45 years of wrist, hip, or rib (4 each, 12 maximum) Age: 3 times first digit of age in years Estrogen use: Never (1) Weight: −1 times weight in lb, divided by 10 and truncated to integer
Weight Criterion		Weight < 70 kg

Study Overview: Analysis of a population-based community sample (CaMos) to assess the diagnostic properties of 4 risk decision rules, compared to the NOF clinical practice guidelines for selecting women for DEXA testing.

Study Intervention: The four decision rules and NOF guidelines evaluated in this analysis are outlined in Table 34.1. Bone mineral density was measured with T scores referenced to Canadian young adult normal values at the femoral neck (Figure 34.1). A T score of < –2.0 served as the treatment threshold, where initiation of pharmacologic therapy was recommended for reduction of postmenopausal fracture incidence.

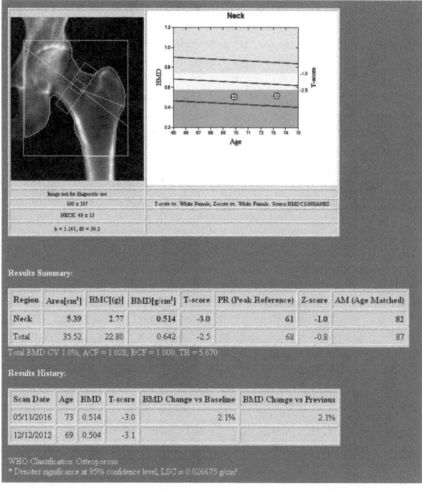

Results Summary:

Region	Area[cm²]	BMC[(g)]	BMD[g/cm²]	T-score	PR (Peak Reference)	Z-score	AM (Age Matched)
Neck	5.39	2.77	0.514	-3.0	61	-1.0	82
Total	35.52	22.80	0.642	-2.5	68	-0.8	87

Total BMD CV 1.0%, ACF = 1.028, BCF = 1.000, TH = 5.670

Results History:

Scan Date	Age	BMD	T-score	BMD Change vs Baseline	BMD Change vs Previous
05/11/2016	73	0.514	-3.0	2.1%	2.1%
12/12/2012	69	0.504	-3.1		

WHO Classification: Osteoporosis
* Denotes significance at 95% confidence level, LSC is 0.026675 g/cm²

Figure 34.1 Dual-energy x-ray absorptiometry (DEXA) image of the left femoral neck demonstrating osteoporosis.

Data Collection: Standardized interview-administered questionnaire, bone mineral density measured by DEXA, body weight measured.

Endpoints: Sensitivity, specificity, and area under the curve for each of the four decision rules and NOF guidelines for identifying women with a T score <−1.0 SD, <−2.0 SD, and ≤−2.5 SD at the femoral neck. Proportion of women recommended for testing, stratified by bone mineral density level and age.

RESULTS

- Percentage of women with T scores of <−1 SD, <−2 SD, and ≤−2.5 SD were 68.3%, 25.4%, and 10.0%, respectively.
- The ORAI and SCORE decision rule had the best performance based on area under the curve for identifying women meeting the treatment threshold (T score <−2.0 SD), yet the body weight criterion had similar AUC for identifying women with osteoporosis (≤−2.5 SD) (see Table 34.2).
- The SCORE, ORAI, and NOF all had high sensitivity for detecting osteoporosis, resulting in >93% of women below the treatment threshold (T score < −2.0) and >96% of women with osteoporosis being recommended for DEXA screening.
- The weight criterion and ABONE (Age, Body Size, No Estrogen) decision rule would miss 13%–17% of women with osteoporosis, but recommend <40% of women with normal bone mineral density for DEXA.

Table 34.2. PERFORMANCE OF DECISION RULES AT THE TREATMENT
THRESHOLD (T SCORE < −2.0 SD)

Decision Rule/ Guideline	Sensitivity % (95% CI)	Specificity % (95% CI)	Area under the Curve (SE)
NOF	93.7 (91.8–95.6)	19.8 (17.9–21.7)	0.67 (0.01)
SCORE	97.5 (96.3–98.8)	20.8 (18.9–22.7)	0.77 (0.01)
ORAI	94.2 (92.3–96.1)	31.9 (29.7–34.1)	0.76 (0.01)
ABONE	79.1 (75.9–82.3)	52.7 (50.3–55.0)	0.71 (0.01)
Weight criterion	79.6 (76.4–82.8)	52.2 (49.9–54.5)	0.74 (0.01)

95% CI = 95% confidence interval, SE = standard error.

Criticisms and Limitations: The study population was composed of white women (96.6%), making generalizability of study results to other racial/ethnic groups not possible. This study provides information from DEXA results at one point in time and does not evaluate the proportion of downstream missed osteoporotic fractures. The actual clinical utility of these decision rules would require prospective assessment in real-world settings.

Other Relevant Studies and Information:

- Identifying women with low bone mineral density using DEXA, along with early pharmacologic intervention, can help reduce incidence of and morbidity associated with osteoporotic fractures.[2,3]
- Both the NOF guidelines and ORAI decision rule suggest that all women ≥65 years old undergo DEXA screening, as these women enter into a period of higher risk for hip fractures.[4]
- The USPSTF recommends DEXA screening for women ≥65 years old and in younger women with fracture risk equal to or greater than that of a 65-year old white woman who has no additional risk factors.[6]
- The USPSTF concluded that there is insufficient evidence to assess the benefits and risks of bone density screening in men.[6]
- A recent systematic review identified the benefit of a newer decision rule, the Osteoporosis Scoring Tool (OST), that is based on age and weight and simple to use as a chart[7] that can be applied with different thresholds for men and women of different ethnic groups.[8]
- The 2004 Surgeon General Report on Bone Health identified the ORAI and OST chart as comparable decision aids for identifying women for DEXA.[9]

Summary and Implications: The ORAI and SCORE decision rules performed the best for targeting DEXA testing among high-risk patients. The ABONE and weight criterion decision rules are comparatively less useful for determining whether women should be screened with DEXA.

CLINICAL CASE: DECISION RULES FOR BONE DENSITY TESTING

Case History:

A 56-year-old postmenopausal, African American female presents to your primary clinic for a general preventive medicine visit. She weighs 180 lb (approximately 81.6 kg) and is in generally good health. She is a current smoker with a 30-year pack history, has not taken any estrogen therapy since her 30s, and has no personal history of minimal trauma fractures. What would you recommend with regard to osteoporosis screening?

Suggested Answer:

Based on this study, the ORAI had the highest accuracy for assessing osteoporosis risk. The patient is >55 years old (5 points), weighs >70 kg (3 points), and is currently not on estrogen therapy (2 points). Thus, the patient reaches the 9-point screening threshold and you should recommend DEXA screening for this patient. Phrased differently, this patient has a risk profile greater than a 65-year-old white woman who has no additional risk factors and should undergo screening under the USPSTF recommendations.

References

1. Cadarette SM, Jaglal SB, Murray TM, McIsaac WJ, Joseph L, Brown JP, for the Canadian Multicentre Osteoporosis Study (CaMos). Evaluation of decision rules for referring women for bone densitometry by dual-energy x-ray absorptiometry. *JAMA*. 2001;286(1):57–63.
2. Genant HK, Cooper C, Poor G, et al. Interim report and recommendations of the World Health Organization task-force for osteoporosis. *Osteporos Int*. 1999;10(4):259–264.
3. Siris ES, Miller PD, Barrett-Connor E, et al. Identification and fracture outcomes of undiagnosed low bone mineral density in postmenopausal women: results from the National Osteoporosis Risk Assessment. *JAMA*. 2001;286(2):2815–2822.
4. Black DM. Screening and treatment in the elderly to reduce osteoporotic fracture risk. *Br J Obstet Gynaecol*. 1996;103 Suppl 13:2–8.
5. Martínez-Aguilà D, Gómez-Vaquero C, Rozadilla A, Romera M, Narváez J, Nolla JM. Decision rules for selecting women for bone mineral density testing: application in postmenopausal women referred to a bone densitometry unit. *J Rheumatol*. 2007;34(6):1307–1312.
6. US Preventive Services Task Force. Screening for osteoporosis: U.S. preventive services task force recommendation statement. *Ann Intern Med*. 2011;154(5):356–364.

7. Cadarette SM, McIsaac WJ, Hawker GA, et al. The validity of decision rules for selecting women with primary osteoporosis for bone mineral density testing. *Osteoporos Int.* 2004;15(5):361–366.

8. Nayak S, Edwards DL, Saleh AA, Greenspan SL. Systematic review and meta-analysis of the performance of clinical risk assessment instruments for screening for osteoporosis or low bone density. *Osteoporos Int.* 2015;26(5):1543–1554.

9. Office of the Surgeon General. Bone health and osteoporosis: A report of the Surgeon General. Rockville, MD: Office of the Surgeon General (US); 2004.

35

Repeat Bone Mineral Density Screening and Osteoporotic Fracture Prediction

CHRISTOPH I. LEE

> ... the current clinical practice of repeating a BMD [bone mineral density] test every 2 years to improve fracture risk stratification may not be necessary in all adults 75 years or older untreated for osteoporosis.
> —Berry et al.[1]

Research Question: Does repeating a BMD screening test within 4 years' time improve fracture risk assessment?

Funding: National Institutes of Health, National Heart, Lung, and Blood Institute's Framingham Heart Study, and Friends of Hebrew SeniorLife.

Year Study Began: 1987

Year Study Published: 2013

Study Location: Framingham, MA.

Who Was Studied: Older men and women from the Framingham Study cohort who had two BMD measures approximately 4 years apart.

Who Was Excluded: Participants with a hip fracture prior to the second BMD test (such individuals are recommended for pharmacologic treatment of osteoporosis regardless of BMD).

How Many Patients: 802

Study Overview: Population-based cohort study involving participants in the Framingham Osteoporosis Study. Clinical characteristics were obtained from the Framingham Study examination closest to the first and second BMD tests. Fracture risk scores were obtained by using the World Health Organization Fracture Risk Assessment Tool (FRAX, version 3.6). The main analysis used Cox proportional hazard models to calculate hazard ratios (HRs) and 95% CIs to determine associations between BMD change and risk of incident major osteoporotic fractures. Unconditional regression models with ROC curves were used to compare models assessing risk of osteoporotic fracture using baseline BMD and BMD changes. A net reclassification index was used to quantify change in risk classification between the first and second BMD measures (high risk = individual with hip fracture risk of ≥3% or major osteoporotic fracture risk of ≥20%; otherwise, low risk).

Study Intervention: Two measures of femoral neck BMD taken up to 4 years apart. The initial measurement occurred between 1987 and 1991 with a dual-photon absorptiometer. Follow-up measurement occurred between 1992 and 1999 with a dual-energy x-ray absorptiometer. The majority (91%) of participants had BMD measures on two different scanners and adjustments were made using cross-calibration of the two scanners.

Follow-Up: Until death, through 2009, or 12 years of follow-up (median follow-up period of 9.6 years).

Endpoints: Primary outcome was hip fracture or major osteoporotic fracture, including fracture of the hip, spine, forearm, or shoulder (Figure 35.1). Other endpoints included the added benefit of BMD change throughout 4 years for osteoporotic fracture risk measurement and change in fracture risk classification after second BMD measure (this latter net reclassification index is an alternative method to describe the clinical contribution of a second BMD measure).

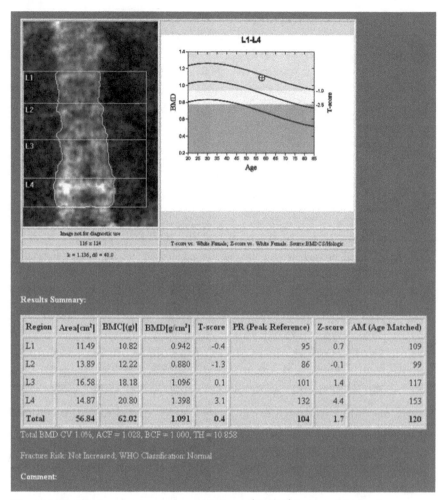

Figure 35.1 Dual-energy x-ray absorptiometry (DEXA) image of the lumbar spine demonstrating a compression fracture at L4, consistent with a diagnosis of osteoporosis.

RESULTS

- Of the 802 participants, 76 (9.5%) experienced an incident hip fracture and 113 (14.1%) experienced a major osteoporotic fracture during the follow-up period. The mean BMD change was –0.6% per year (with a SD of 1.8%) (Table 35.1).

- After adjusting for clinical characteristics and baseline BMD, annual percent BMD change per SD decrease was associated with both higher hip fracture risk (HR, 1.43; 95% CI, 1.16–1.78) and higher major osteoporotic fracture risk (HR, 1.21; 95% CI, 1.01–1.45).
- Adding BMD change to a model with baseline BMD did not improve performance on the ROC curve (AUC 0.71, 95% CI, 0.65–0.78 for the baseline BMD model, vs. AUC 0.68, 95% CI, 0.62–0.75, for the BMD percent change model).

Table 35.1. CHANGE IN RISK CLASSIFICATION FROM FIRST TO SECOND BMD MEASURE

	Fracture during Follow-up	No Fracture during Follow-up
Net reclassification index for hip fractures,[a] %, 95% CI	3.9 (–2.2 to 9.9)	–2.2 (–4.5 to 0.1)
Net reclassification index for major osteoporotic fractures,[a] %, 95% CI	9.7 (3.4 to 15.7)	–4.6 (–6.7 to –2.6)

[a] Participants were classified as high risk for hip fracture if ≥3% fracture risk score and high risk for major osteoporotic fracture if ≥20% fracture risk score.

Criticisms and Limitations: The majority of participants had BMD measured on two different machines, making misclassification errors possible. There was no confirmation of major osteoporotic fractures by using medical records; thus, some of the associated outcomes may have been misclassified. With the exception of estrogen, there was no data on the use of bisphosphonates or other osteoporosis medications. Given the timing of this study, most participants were probably untreated for osteoporosis, and the results may not generalize to a treated population. The study population was mostly white, making generalizability to other racial/ethnic groups difficult. Finally, many frail, elderly Framingham study patients did not return to have multiple measures of BMD and were excluded from this analysis.

Other Relevant Studies and Information:

- The World Health Organization Fracture Risk Assessment Tool (FRAX) estimates the 10-year absolute risk of hip and major osteoporotic fracture based on individual risk factors, with or without BMD measures.[2]
- The FRAX risk score is applicable to postmenopausal women and men 40–90 years of age. The National Osteoporosis Foundation Clinician's

Guide recommends treating patients with FRAX 10-year risk scores of ≥3% for hip fracture or ≥20% for major osteoporotic fracture.[3]

- Currently, in the United States, most older individuals undergo serial BMD tests at an average of 2.2-year intervals.[4]
- The Study on Osteoporotic Fracture (SOF) found that <10% of postmenopausal women with mild osteopenia or normal BMD end up losing bone density to osteoporotic levels within 15 years.[5]
- The USPSTF recommends BMD screening for women aged ≥65 years and in younger women with fracture risk equal to or greater than that of a 65-year-old white woman who has no additional risk factors.[6]
- The USPSTF recommends waiting a minimum of 2 years to obtain a second BMD measure using DEXA but also notes that waiting longer periods in between tests may improve future risk prediction.[6]

Summary and Implications: A repeat BMD test within 4 years adds little additional value beyond the baseline BMD test when assessing hip fracture risk. Moreover, a repeat test within 4 years may not improve fracture risk stratification used for clinical management of osteoporosis.

CLINICAL CASE: NEED FOR REPEAT BONE DENSITY TESTING

Case History:

A 67-year-old female presents to your primary care clinic for a routine preventive clinic visit. She is in good health and is currently only taking one medication to treat her mild hypertension. Her last DEXA scan was 2 years prior when she had a T-score of –2.0, suggesting osteopenia. Her WHO FRAX 10-year risk scores were 1.1% for hip fracture and 8.7% for major osteoporotic fracture. The patient is concerned about not being on preventive medications like her friends are, and wonders if she should have a repeat DEXA scan. How should you advise this patient?

Suggested Answer:

While on average most older Americans are getting serial DEXA scans about every 2 years, this study suggests that a second BMD test within 4 years' time is unlikely to change clinical management, especially among individuals with mild bone loss at baseline (mild osteopenia). Under USPSTF guidelines, this patient does qualify to receive a repeat DEXA. However, there is likely little added value from a repeat test after just 2 years from her baseline test, and you should inform the patient that there would likely be no clinical management change based on a repeat DEXA scan at this time.

References

1. Berry SD, Samelson EJ, Pencina MJ, etc. Repeat bone mineral density screening and prediction of hip and major osteoporotic fracture. *JAMA*. 2013;310(12):1256–1262.
2. Kanis JA, McCloskey EV, Johansson H, Strom O, Borgstrom F, Oden A; National Osteoporosis Guideline Group. Case finding for the management of osteoporosis with FRAX—assessment and intervention thresholds for the UK. *Osteoporos Int*. 2008;19(10):1395–1408.
3. Siris ES, Baim S, Nattiv A. Primary care use of FRAX: absolute fracture risk assessment in postmenopausal women and older men. *Postgrad Med*. 2010;122(1):82–90.
4. McAdam-Marx C, Unni S, Ye X, Nelson S, Nickman NA. Effect of Medicare reimbursement reduction for imaging services on osteoporosis screening rates. *J Am Geriatr Soc*. 2012;60(3):511–516.
5. Gourlay ML, Fine JP, Preisser JS, et al; Study of Osteoporotic Fractures Research Group. Bone-density testing interval and transition to osteoporosis in older women. *N Engl J Med*. 2012;366(3):225–233.
6. US Preventive Services Task Force. Screening for osteoporosis: U.S. preventive services task force recommendation statement. *Ann Intern Med*. 2011; 154(5):356–364.

36

Ultrasound for Diagnosing Suspected Symptomatic Deep Venous Thrombosis

CHRISTOPH I. LEE

... both serial 2-point ultrasonography plus D-dimer and whole-leg color-coded Doppler ultrasonography represent reliable diagnostic options for the management of symptomatic patients with suspected DVT of the lower extremities.

—BERNARDI ET AL.[1]

Research Question: Is serial 2-point ultrasonography (proximal veins) plus D-dimer comparable to whole-leg color-coded Doppler ultrasonography for diagnosing suspected symptomatic deep venous thrombosis (DVT)?

Funding: SISET (Società Italiana per lo Studio dell'Emostasi e della Trombosi). D-dimer testing kits provided free of charge by AGEN Biomedical Ltd.

Year Study Began: 2003

Year Study Published: 2008

Study Location: 14 Italian universities and civic hospitals.

Who Was Studied: All consecutive adult outpatients referred by the emergency department or a primary care physician with a first episode of suspected DVT of the lower extremities.

Who Was Excluded: Patients <18 years of age; pregnant; or with a history of venous thromboembolism, life expectancy <3 months, or ongoing anticoagulation (>48 hours), mandatory anticoagulation indication (e.g., atrial fibrillation), or geographic inaccessibility to follow-up.

How Many Patients: 2,098

Study Overview: Prospective randomized multicenter study. Patients were assigned to either the 2-point or whole-leg ultrasound strategy. Patients with normal 2-point ultrasound underwent D-dimer testing. If D-dimer was normal (no visible agglutination), then patients were spared anticoagulation. If D-dimer was abnormal (visible agglutination or noninterpretable findings), then patients were scheduled for a repeat 2-point ultrasound within 1 week. Patients with normal repeat ultrasound findings were spared anticoagulation.

Study Intervention: Patients were randomized to either 2-point ultrasound (proximal veins only, n = 1,045) or whole-leg ultrasound (n = 1,053). The 2-point ultrasound strategy involved using a 5–10 MHz linear probe with compression at the common femoral vein at the groin and the popliteal vein at the popliteal fossa. Whole-leg ultrasound utilized color Doppler technology to evaluate the entire deep venous system, from the groin to the ankle (no compression beyond the proximal veins). Compression was used as the only diagnostic criterion to diagnose DVT in both study arms. Physicians experienced in vascular ultrasound performed all diagnostic evaluations.

Follow-Up: Three-month follow-up interview, physical examination, and/or ultrasound for patients with normal ultrasound findings.

Endpoints: Incidence of symptomatic DVT in patients spared anticoagulation therapy on the basis of a normal initial workup with either serial 2-point ultrasonography plus D-dimer or whole-leg Doppler ultrasonography.

RESULTS

- The observed difference in symptomatic DVT at 3 months follow-up between the two groups was 0.3% (95% CI, –1.4% to 0.8%).

This difference was within the predetermined equivalence limit (Table 36.1).

- Despite a higher initial prevalence of DVT in the whole-leg ultrasound group (absolute difference, 4.3%; 95% CI, 0.5%–8.1%), outcomes were similar between the two groups. The difference in initial prevalence was entirely accounted for by isolated calf DVTs identified during whole-leg ultrasound.
- Sensitivity analyses accounting for patients who died or were lost to follow-up during the study period did not yield different results from the main analysis.

Table 36.1. THE TRIAL'S KEY FINDINGS

Outcome	2-Point Ultrasound Strategy	Whole-Leg Ultrasound Strategy
Initial prevalence of DVT		
% (no./total)	22.1% (231/1,045)	26.4% (278/1,053)
[95% CI]	[19.6%–24.6%]	[23.7%–29.1%]
Incidence of symptomatic DVT at 3 months		
% (no./total)	0.9% (7/801)	1.2% (9/763)
[95% CI]	[0.3%–1.8%]	[0.5%–2.2%]

Criticisms and Limitations: The majority of follow-up (approximately 75%) was conducted by telephone rather than clinic visits (approximately 25%). Compression ultrasonography limitations include the need for serial tests if the first ultrasound is negative, and missed isolated thrombi in the iliac veins or proximal portions of the femoral veins.

Other Relevant Studies and Information:

- The major difference between the 2-point ultrasound strategy and whole-leg ultrasound strategy is that the latter evaluates the calf veins. However, since the ultimate incidence of symptomatic DVT at 3 months was similar between groups, the clinical relevance of calf DVTs is called into question.
- Previous studies have also suggested the equivocal significance of calf DVTs and the need for evaluation of calf veins in suspected cases of lower extremity DVTs.[2,3]
- This study found that, in symptomatic outpatients, proximal DVT always involved the common femoral vein, the popliteal vein, or

both; thus, similar to findings in prior studies, this trial suggests that investigation of the superficial and deep femoral veins may not be necessary in cases of suspected lower extremity DVTs.[4,5]

- A meta-analysis of 7 studies examining 3-month incidence of DVT after a negative whole-leg compression ultrasound found a combined DVT incidence of 0.57% (95% CI, 0.25%–0.89%) across studies.[6]

- The American Academy of Family Physicians (AAFP) and the American College of Physicians (ACP) clinical practice guidelines suggest the following approach: (1) In patients with a low pretest probability of DVT according to the Wells score, ultrasound (2-point or whole-leg) is not needed unless the D-dimer is positive or unavailable. (2) Ultrasound (2-point or whole-leg) is recommended for patients with intermediate to high pretest probability of DVT based on the Wells score. Repeat ultrasound may be required for those with suspected calf vein DVT and a negative initial ultrasound investigation.[7]

Summary and Implications: Whole-leg ultrasonography with color Doppler requires top-quality ultrasound equipment and experienced operators. The more limited, 2-point DVT ultrasound strategy can be performed with older equipment and with minimal training. This study demonstrated that 2-point ultrasonography is equivalent to the whole-leg ultrasonography for diagnosing symptomatic DVT.

CLINICAL CASE: SUSPECTED DEEP VENOUS THROMBOSIS

Case History:

A 68-year-old male who was recently bedridden after hip replacement 2 weeks ago presents to the urgent care facility after hours with localized tenderness in his left upper leg. He has no swelling or pitting edema in the symptomatic leg on physical exam. He has no history of cancer or other significant comorbidities. You order a D-dimer that comes back as indeterminate. Since it's after hours, no dedicated vascular sonographer is on duty, and the night-shift radiology technologist can only perform a standard 2-point lower extremity ultrasound. Is an ultrasound necessary? If so, then should you keep the patient in the observation unit until the morning for a whole-leg ultrasound, or proceed with the 2-point lower extremity ultrasound to rule out DVT?

Suggested Answer:

Based on his Wells score of 2 points (a point each for being recently bedridden and having localized tenderness in the deep venous system), this patient is at moderate probability for DVT. Thus, based on AAFP and ACP practice guidelines, a diagnostic ultrasound is warranted. Bernardi et al.[1] found that 2-point ultrasound with compression is as accurate as whole-leg ultrasound with color Doppler in diagnosing symptomatic DVT (Figure 36.1). You should not delay diagnostic workup by waiting for a whole-leg ultrasound and should triage the patient based on the 2-point ultrasound findings.

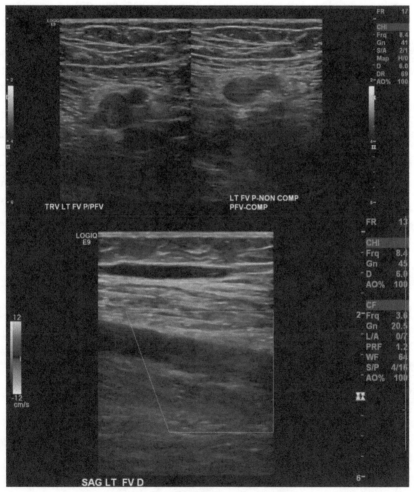

Figure 36.1 Grayscale (top) and color Doppler (bottom) ultrasound images of the left femoral artery demonstrating noncompressibility of the vein (top) and significantly reduced blood flow (bottom), consistent with deep venous thrombosis (DVT).

References

1. Bernardi E, Camporese G, Büller HR, et al. Serial 2-point ultrasonography plus D-dimer vs whole-leg color-coded Doppler ultrasonography for diagnosing suspected symptomatic deep vein thrombosis: a randomized controlled trial. *JAMA*. 2008;300(14):1653–1659.

2. Kearon C, Ginsberg JS, Douketis J, et al. A randomized trial of diagnostic strategies after normal proximal vein ultrasonography for suspected deep venous thrombosis: D-dimer testing compared with repeated ultrasonography. *Ann Intern Med*. 2005;142(7):490–496.

3. Stevens SM, Elliott CG, Chan KJ, Egger MJ, Ahmed KM. Withholding anticoagulation after a negative result on duplex ultrasonography for suspected symptomatic deep venous thrombosis. *Ann Intern Med*. 2004;140(12):985–991.

4. Lensing AW, Prandoni P, Brandjes D, et al. Detection of deep-vein thrombosis by real-time B-mode ultrasonography. *N Engl J Med*. 1989;320(6):342–345.

5. Cogo A, Lensing AWA, Prandoni P, Hirsh J. Distribution of thrombosis in patients with symptomatic deep vein thrombosis: implications for simplifying the diagnostic process with compression ultrasound. *Arch Intern Med*. 1993;153(24):2777–2780.

6. Johnson SA, Stevens SM, Woller SC, et al. Risk of deep vein thrombosis following a single negative whole-leg compression ultrasound: a systematic review and meta-analysis. *JAMA*. 2010;303(5):438–445.

7. Qaseem A, Snow V, Barry P, et al. Current diagnosis of venous thromboembolism in primary care: a clinical practice guideline from the American Academy of Family Physicians and the American College of Physicians. *Ann Intern Med*. 2007;146(6):454–458.

Cancer Screening and Management

37

The Cochrane Review of Screening Mammography

MICHAEL E. HOCHMAN

> For every 2000 women invited for screening throughout 10 years, one will have her life prolonged . . . [and] 10 healthy women who would not have had a breast cancer diagnosis if there had not been screening will be diagnosed as cancer patients, and will be treated unnecessarily.
>
> —GØTZSCHE AND NIELSEN[1]

Research Question: Is screening mammography effective?[1]

Funding: The Cochrane Collaboration, an independent, nonprofit organization supported by governments, universities, hospital trusts, charities, and donations. The Cochrane Collaboration does not accept commercial funding.

Year Study Began: The earliest trial began in 1963 and the most recent began in 1991.

Year Study Published: The results of the individual trials were published during the 1970s, 1980s, 1990s, and 2000s. This Cochrane review was published in 2011.

Study Location: The trials were conducted in Sweden, the United States, Canada, and the United Kingdom.

Study Overview: This was a meta-analysis of randomized clinical trials of screening mammography in women without previously diagnosed breast cancer.

Which Trials Were Included: A total of 11 randomized trials were identified using an exhaustive search strategy; however, 3 were not eligible for inclusion because of methodological limitations and 1 was excluded due to bias. Therefore, seven trials were included in the meta-analysis. These trials are listed with the country and start date in parentheses:

- The Health Insurance Plan trial (USA 1963)
- The Malmö trial (Sweden 1978)
- The Two-County trial (Sweden 1977)
- The Canadian trials (2 trials with different age groups; Canada 1980)
- The Stockholm trial (Sweden 1981)
- The Göteborg trial (Sweden 1982)
- The United Kingdom age trial (United Kingdom 1991)

Study Intervention: In all 7 trials, women were randomized to receive either an invitation for breast cancer screening with mammography (Figure 37.1) or no invitation for screening. Women in the screening group were invited for 2–9 rounds of screening, depending on the trial.

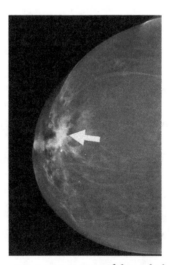

Figure 37.1 CC view screening mammogram of the right breast with a spiculated mass at anterior depth that is concerning for breast carcinoma (arrow), requiring additional evaluation (BIRADS 0).

RESULTS

See Table 37.1 for a summary of key findings over 13 years of follow-up.

- Data were available for 599,090 women over 13 years of follow-up.
- The authors judged 3 of the 7 trials to have optimal randomization methodology; for these three trials, data were available for 292,153 women.
- Screening mammography appeared to reduce breast cancer mortality but not all-cause mortality.

Table 37.1. SUMMARY OF KEY FINDINGS, 13 YEARS OF FOLLOW-UP

Outcome	Relative Risk with Screening (95% Confidence Intervals)
Breast Cancer Mortality	
All 7 trials	0.81 (0.74–0.87)
3 trials with optimal methodology	0.90 (0.79–1.02)
All-Cause Mortality	
All 7 trials	Unreliable[a]
3 trials with optimal methodology	0.99 (0.95–1.03)
Surgeries[b]	
All 7 trials	1.35 (1.26–1.44)
3 trials with optimal methodology	1.31 (1.22–1.44)
Radiotherapy	
All 7 trials	1.32 (1.16–1.50)
3 trials with optimal methodology	1.24 (1.04–1.49)

[a] The authors felt this number was unreliable, and therefore do not report it.
[b] Mastectomies and lumpectomies.

Criticisms and Limitations: Many of the individual trials included in this meta-analysis suffered from methodological flaws. Some of these flaws may have biased the results in favor of the screening group while others may have biased the results in favor of the controls:

- In many cases women assigned to the control groups appeared to be systematically different from those assigned to the screening groups. For example, in the Two-County trial more women in the control group than in the screening group had been diagnosed with breast cancer prior to the start of the trial. Differences such as these may have biased the results.

- Determination of breast cancer mortality rates in many of the trials was potentially biased or inaccurate. The physicians who determined the cause of death for study subjects were frequently aware of whether the subjects had been assigned to the screening versus control groups, and it is possible that their judgments were influenced by this knowledge. Furthermore, few autopsies of patients who died were performed, and therefore many of the cause-of-death determinations may have been inaccurate.

- Some experts have criticized the screening mammography trials because, particularly in some of the trials, women in the control groups began receiving screening before the trials were concluded. Because it presumably takes several years before the benefits of screening are apparent, it is unlikely this would have substantially affected the trial results. Still, it is possible that mammograms among controls partially obscured the benefits of screening.

- Some women in these trials received one-view mammograms rather than the standard two-view studies. It is possible that the one-view films were less effective at identifying cancers.

- These trials were all conducted several years ago. Breast cancer treatments have improved in recent years, and some experts believe that with current treatment options, the benefits of early detection of breast cancer may be smaller.[2]

Other Relevant Studies and Information:

- A recent modeling study suggests that screening mammography every 2 years "achieves most of the benefit of annual screening with less harm." In addition, this study suggests that screening mammograms in women between the ages of 40–49 lead to only a small benefit but a high rate of false-positive results.[3]

- Table 37.2 lists breast cancer screening guidelines from two major organizations.

Summary and Implications: Most of the trials of screening mammography have considerable methodological flaws. Despite these limitations, the Cochrane Review suggests that screening mammography modestly reduces breast cancer mortality but may not reduce all-cause mortality. In addition, screening mammography leads to the diagnosis and unnecessary treatment of a substantial number of women who may never have developed symptoms of breast cancer. According to the authors, for every 2,000

Table 37.2. MAJOR BREAST CANCER SCREENING GUIDELINES

Guideline	Recommendations
The US Preventive Services Task Force	• Screening recommended every 2 years for women 50–74 years of age • "the decision to start [screening] before the age of 50 years should be an individual one and take patient context into account . . ."
The American Cancer Society	• Yearly mammograms are recommended starting at age 40 and continuing for as long as a woman is in good health

women offered screening mammograms over a 10-year period, 1 will have her life prolonged while 10 will be treated for breast cancer unnecessarily. The appropriate use of screening mammography remains an area of considerable controversy.

CLINICAL CASE: SCREENING MAMMOGRAPHY

Case History:

A 68-year-old woman with chronic obstructive pulmonary disease, diabetes, and osteoporosis visits your clinic for a routine visit. When you mention that she is due for a screening mammogram, she protests: "I have so many other medical problems. Why do we need to look for more?"

Based on the results of the Cochrane Review on mammography, what can you tell this patient about the risks and benefits of screening mammography?

Suggested Answer:

The Cochrane Mammography review suggests that screening mammography modestly reduces breast cancer mortality but may not reduce all-cause mortality. In addition, screening mammography leads to the diagnosis and unnecessary treatment of a substantial number of women who may never have developed symptoms of breast cancer. Some women may not feel that this trade-off is worth it.

The woman in this vignette has other significant comorbidities, and does not want to "look for more." Thus, it would be perfectly reasonable for her to opt not to undergo screening. Since this patient is in poor health, screening may not even be appropriate for her since the benefits of screening occur several years down the road and she may not live long enough to realize these benefits. Indeed, the American Cancer Society only recommends screening among women in good overall health.

References

1. Gøtzsche PC, Nielsen M. Screening for breast cancer with mammography. *Cochrane Database Syst Rev.* 2011;1:CD001877.
2. Welch HG. Screening mammography—a long run for a short slide? *N Engl J Med.* 2010;363(13):1276–1278.
3. Mandelblatt JS et al. Effects of mammography screening under different screening schedules: model estimates of potential benefits and harms. *Ann Intern Med.* 2009;151:738–747.

38

Breast Cancer Screening in Average-Risk Women

CHRISTOPH I. LEE

Our meta-analysis of mammography screening trials indicates breast cancer mortality benefit for all age groups from 39 to 69 years, with insufficient data for older women. False-positive results are common in all age groups and lead to additional imaging and biopsies. Women aged 40 to 49 years experience the highest rate of additional imaging, whereas their biopsy rate is lower than that for older women. Mammography screening at any age is a tradeoff of a continuum of benefits and harms. The ages at which this tradeoff becomes acceptable to individuals and society are not clearly resolved by the available evidence.

—NELSON ET AL.[1]

Primary Research Question: What is the effectiveness of mammography screening in decreasing breast cancer mortality among average-risk women aged 40–49 years and ≥70 years, and what are the harms of screening with mammography?

Funding: Agency for Healthcare Research and Quality.

Year Study Began: The earliest trial began in 1963 and the most recent trial began in 1991.

Year Study Published: Relevant published trials and other data sources (including the Breast Cancer Surveillance Consortium) available through 2008 were included in the analysis. This systematic review was published in 2009.

Study Location: The included randomized controlled trials were conducted in Sweden, the United States, Canada, and the United Kingdom.

Study Overview: This was a systematic review and meta-analysis of the existing evidence performed for the US Preventive Services Task Force (USPSTF) to aid in determining their revised recommendations for population-based breast cancer screening. This analysis aimed to fill evidence gaps that were unresolved at the time of the 2002 USPSTF recommendation.

Which Trials Were Included: Screening mammography, clinical breast examination, and breast self-examination effectiveness data were abstracted from randomized controlled trials and updates to previously published trials that included mortality outcomes data. Data on harms of screening were obtained from published studies, meta-analyses, and primary data from the Breast Cancer Surveillance Consortium (BCSC), a collaboration of breast imaging registries across the United States.

Study Interventions: The main intervention examined was screening mammography; other interventions included clinical breast examination and breast self-examination.

Endpoints: The effectiveness and harms of screening mammography for decreasing breast cancer mortality among average-risk women aged 40–49 and ≥70 years. In addition, effectiveness and harms of clinical breast examination and breast self-examination as methods of cancer screening for all age groups.

RESULTS

- Based on 8 randomized trials, screening mammography reduces breast cancer mortality by 15% for women aged 39–49 years (relative risk = 0.85 [95% CI, 0.75–0.96]). Number need to invite to prevent 1 breast cancer death and relative risks for other age groups can be found in Table 38.1.
- Data for women ≥70 years were confined to the Swedish Two-County trial of women aged 70–74 years, which demonstrated a relative risk for breast cancer mortality of 1.12 (95% CI, 0.73–1.72) based on a conservative determination of cause of death.

- Based on BCSC data, women aged 40–49 years experienced the highest false-positive screening rate (97.8/1,000 women per screening round) and the highest rate of additional imaging (84.3/1,000 women per screening round), but the lowest false-negative rate (1.0/1,000 women per screening round). While rates of additional imaging decreased with age, biopsy rates increased with age.
- Rates of overdiagnosis (breast cancer detected on screening that would not have led to clinically significant disease during a patient's lifetime) varied from <1% to 30%, with most between 1% and 10% of all screen-detected cancers.
- Trials for breast self-examination have shown increased benign biopsy rates and no reductions in mortality, whereas the incremental effectiveness of clinical breast examination in addition to screening mammography has not been proven in large, well-designed trials.

Table 38.1. MORTALITY RELATIVE RISKS FROM SCREENING TRIALS BY AGE

Age Group (Years)	Number of RCTs Included	RR for Breast Cancer Mortality Value (95% CI)	NNI to Prevent 1 Cancer Death Value (95% CI)
39–49	8	0.85 (0.75–0.96)	1,904 (929–6,378)
50–59	6	0.86 (0.75–0.99)	1,339 (322–7,455)
60–69	2	0.68 (0.54–0.87)	377 (230–1,050)
70–74	1	1.12 (0.73–1.72)	Not available

RCT = randomized controlled trial; RR = relative risk; NNI = number needed to invite to screening.

Criticisms and Limitations: Estimates of benefits and harms of screening in this analysis are based heavily on screen-film mammography, which is not the current technology in use (>95% of US mammography units are now digital). No definitive studies regarding appropriate intervals for mammography screening were identified, and the available evidence has not resolved the ages at which the tradeoff between benefits and harms are acceptable.

Other Relevant Studies and Information:

- This systematic review partly influenced the USPSTF recommendation revision for screening mammography in 2009. Previously, in 2002, the USPSTF had recommended mammography screening, with or without clinical breast examination, every 1–2 years for women aged ≥40 years.[2]

- The USPSTF recommends that the decision to start regular screening mammography before age 50 be an individual one, taking into account the patient's values regarding specific benefits and harms. The USPSTF concluded that the current evidence is insufficient to make recommendations for women >74 years old.[3]
- The American Cancer Society (ACS) and the American College of Radiology (ACR) recommend annual screening mammography for women aged ≥40 years, and that they continue to do so for as long as they are in good health.[4,5]

Summary and Implications: Meta-analysis of available trial data demonstrates a 15% mortality reduction among women aged 39–49 years with routine screening mammography. This age group has the highest rates of additional imaging but lowest rates of benign biopsy. There is currently little data available regarding the screening benefits and harms for women aged ≥70 years, which represents the fastest growing population in the United States.

CLINICAL CASE: MAMMOGRAPHY SCREENING AMONG OLDER WOMEN

Case History:
A 75-year-old female presents to your primary care clinic for a routine checkup and to refill her prescriptions. She is interested in discussing the need for screening mammography at her age, and would like to get your opinion on the matter. She is in relatively good health except for mild hypertension and hyperlipidemia. She is an active golfer and travels often. How should you advise her?

Suggested Answer:
Based on the current randomized controlled trial data, there is not enough high-quality information to recommend for or against routine mammography screening among older women. The USPSTF leaves this decision to be made by patients with input from their physicians, and weighing their own preferences with regards to potential benefits and harms. The ACS and ACR recommend routine screening for all older women in good health, even if they are older than age 70 (Figure 38.1). For this patient, comorbidities do not seem to be an issue, and you should engage in a discussion with her in order to get a sense of her personal values with regard to potential benefits and harms of continued routine screening.

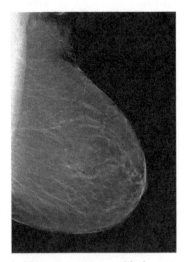

Figure 38.1 Mediolateral oblique image in an elderly patient with breasts that consist almost entirely of fat. The craniocaudal image was equally unremarkable. No suspicious abnormality is identified.

References

1. Nelson HD, Tyne K, Naik A, Bougatsos C, Chan BK, Humphrey L; US Preventive Services Task Force. Screening for breast cancer: an update for the U.S. Preventive Services Task Force. *Ann Intern Med.* 2009;151(10):727–737.
2. US Preventive Services Task Force. Screening for breast cancer: recommendations and rationale. *Ann Intern Med.* 2002;137(5 Part 1):344–346.
3. US Preventive Services Task Force. Screening for breast cancer: U.S. Preventive Services Task Force recommendation statement. *Ann Intern Med.* 2009;151(10):716–726.
4. American Cancer Society. American Cancer Society recommendations for early breast cancer detection in women without breast symptoms. http://www.cancer.org/cancer/breastcancer/moreinformation/breastcancerearlydetection/breast-cancer-early-detection-acs-recs. Revised October 20, 2015. Accessed May 30, 2015.
5. Lee CH, Dershaw DD, Kopans D, et al. Breast cancer screening with imaging: recommendations from the Society of Breast Imaging and the ACR on the use of mammography, breast MRI, breast ultrasound, and other technologies for the detection of clinically occult breast cancer. *J Am Coll Radiol.* 2010;7(1):18–27.

39

Efficacy of Screening Breast MRI for High-Risk Women

The Dutch MRI Screening (MRISC) Study

CHRISTOPH I. LEE

> ... our study shows that the screening program we used, especially MRI screening, can detect breast cancer at an early stage in women at risk for breast cancer.
>
> —KRIEGE ET AL.[1]

Research Question: Does screening including MRI facilitate the early diagnosis of breast cancer among high-risk women?

Funding: Dutch Health Insurance Council.

Year Study Began: 1999

Year Study Published: 2004

Study Location: Six familial-cancer clinics in the Netherlands.

Who Was Studied: Women aged 25–70 years with a cumulative lifetime risk of breast cancer of ≥15% due to familial or genetic predisposition.

Who Was Excluded: Women with symptoms suggestive of breast cancer or personal history of breast cancer.

How Many Patients: 1,909

Study Overview: Prospective cohort study of high-risk women who attend 1 of the 6 participating Dutch family cancer clinics for screening. For analysis, women were divided into three risk groups: BRCA or other mutation carriers (50%–85% cumulative lifetime risk), a high-risk group (30%–49%), and a moderate-risk group (15%–29%).

Exposures: Women were screened every 6 months with a clinical breast examination performed by an experienced physician and annually by mammography and MRI interpreted by experienced radiologists. A dynamic gadolinium contrast-enhanced breast MRI was performed using a standard protocol, between days 5 and 15 of the menstrual cycle. The results of the mammography and MRI were not linked in order to blind each examination result.

Follow-Up: Median follow-up period of 2.9 years (mean 2.7, range 0.1–3.9 years).

Endpoints: Sensitivity, specificity, and positive predictive value of screening mammography or screening MRI relative to one another. The AUC for the 2 imaging methods was used as an index for the inherent capacity of a screening method to discriminate between positive and negative cases. Tumor characteristics were compared with those in two age-matched control groups from a national registry and a large prospective study.

RESULTS

- The overall rate of breast cancer detection was 9.5 per 1,000 woman-years at risk (95% CI, 7.1%–12.3%), with the highest rate (26.5/1,000) among mutation carriers.
- MRI detected 32/45 breast cancers (22 not visible on mammography) and missed 13/45 breast cancers (8 visible on mammography, 4 interval cancers, and 1 detected by clinical exam alone) (Table 39.1).
- Mammography detected 18/45 breast cancers (10 visible on MRI) and missed 27/45 breast cancers (22 visible on MRI, 4 interval cancers, and 1 detected by clinical exam alone).

- The AUC was 0.686 for mammography and 0.827 for MRI (difference 0.141; 95% CI, 0.020–0.262; $P < 0.05$).
- The proportion of tumors ≤10 mm in size was significantly greater in the MRI screening group (43.2%) than in either control group (14.0%, $P < 0.001$ and 12.5%, $P = 0.04$).
- The incidence of lymph node metastases (node-positive and micrometastases) was 21.4% in the MRI screening group, compared to 52.4% ($P < 0.001$) and 56.4% ($P = 0.001$) in the 2 control groups.
- Screening MRI led to twice as many unnecessary diagnostic examinations as did mammography (420 vs. 207) and 3 times as many unnecessary benign biopsies (24 vs. 7).

Table 39.1. THE STUDY'S KEY FINDINGS

Screening Method	Sensitivity[a]	Specificity	PPV
Clinical breast examination	17.9%	98.1%	9.6%[b]
Mammography	33.3%	95.0%	8.0%[c]
MRI	79.5%	89.9%	7.1%[d]

PPV = positive predictive value.
[a] For invasive breast cancer.
[b] Among 83 clinical breast examinations judged as probably benign or suspicious.
[c] Among 225 mammograms with BI-RADS assessments ≥3.
[d] Among 452 MRI screenings with BI-RADS assessments ≥3.

Criticisms and Limitations: One of the control groups used was from a national registry with no detailed family history or screening information. Beyond diagnostic capability and workup to tissue diagnosis, this study does not provide information regarding improved patient outcomes from MRI screening.

Other Relevant Studies and Information:

- Combined breast MRI and mammography screening has higher sensitivity than combined ultrasound and mammography screening (92.7% vs. 52%) among high-risk women.[2]
- Microsimulation modeling work suggests that screening MRI is cost-effective for high-risk women, and that the cost-effectiveness increases with increasing risk.[3]
- The American Cancer Society recommends annual MRI and mammography for women with a lifetime risk of breast cancer >20% according to risk assessment tools. For women with 15%–20% lifetime

risk, the American Cancer Society states that there is not enough evidence to make a recommendation for or against yearly MRI screening.[4]

- The American College of Radiology considers breast MRI screening usually appropriate among high-risk women (≥20% lifetime risk, score 9 out of 9) and among intermediate-risk women (15%–20% lifetime risk, score 7 out of 9).[5]

Summary and Implications: Breast MRI screening has higher sensitivity than mammography for high-risk women, but both the specificity and positive predictive value are lower than for mammography screening. MRI screening also appears to improve the chance of diagnosing breast cancer at an early stage compared with the distribution of tumor staging in two external control groups.

CLINICAL CASE: BREAST MRI SCREENING IN HIGH-RISK WOMEN

Case History:

A 50-year-old female presents to your primary care clinic to discuss starting routine mammography screening. She informs you that her mother had breast cancer at age 64 and her sister was recently diagnosed with breast cancer at age 46. Her age of menarche was 12 years old, and she has had one child at age 24. She is currently asymptomatic and has scheduled a screening mammogram next week. Would you recommend screening MRI as well as a mammogram for this patient?

Suggested Answer:

Multiple risk assessment tools are available, including the modified Gail Model, Tyrer-Cuzick calculator, and the Breast Cancer Surveillance Consortium 5-year risk calculator. The National Cancer Institute offers an online risk assessment tool (http://www.cancer.gov/BCRISKTOOL/). Given the fact that the patient has 2 first-degree relatives with diagnosed breast cancer, she has >20% lifetime risk of breast cancer (Figure 39.1). Based on the Dutch MRI screening study, this patient would benefit from screening MRI for detecting breast cancer at earlier stages. However, she should be informed of the potential increased risks of unnecessary diagnostic workups and benign biopsies if she chooses to undergo MRI screening.

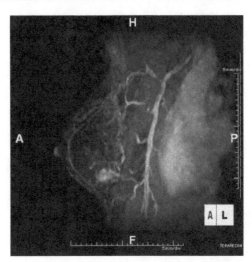

Figure 39.1 Contrast enhanced fat-saturated and subtracted T1 3D image reconstruction of the right breast in a woman with dense breast tissue and multiple risk factors for breast cancer who presented for screening MRI. Note the area of suspicious abnormal focal enhancement within the inferior breast tissue. This appeared as an area of linear non–mass-like enhancement at 6:00 on axial images.

References

1. Kriege M, Brekelmans CT, Boetes C, et al. Efficacy of MRI and mammography for breast cancer screening in women with a familial or genetic predisposition. *N Engl J Med*. 2004;351(5):427–437.
2. Berg WA. Tailored supplemental screening for breast cancer: what now and what next? *AJR Am J Roentgenol*. 2009;192(2):390–399.
3. Plevritis SK, Kurian AW, Sigal BM, et al. Cost-effectiveness of screening BRCA1/2 mutation carriers with breast magnetic resonance imaging. *JAMA*. 2006;295(20):2374–2384.
4. American Cancer Society. American Cancer Society recommendations for early breast cancer detection in women without breast symptoms. http://www.cancer.org/cancer/breastcancer/moreinformation/breastcancerearlydetection/breast-cancer-early-detection-acs-recs. Revised October 20, 2015. Accessed May 30, 2015.
5. American College of Radiology. ACR appropriateness criteria—breast cancer screening. http://www.acr.org/~/media/ACR/Documents/AppCriteria/Diagnostic/BreastCancerScreening.pdf. Published 2012. Accessed May 30, 2015.

40

Performance of Digital versus Screen-Film Mammography

The Digital Mammography Imaging Screening Trial (DMIST)

CHRISTOPH I. LEE

We found that digital mammography was significantly better than conventional film mammography at detecting breast cancer in young women, premenopausal and perimenopausal women, and women with dense breasts.

—PISANO ET AL.[1]

Research Question: Is digital mammography more effective than screen-film mammography for breast cancer screening?

Funding: National Cancer Institute.

Year Study Began: 2001

Year Study Published: 2005

Study Location: 33 sites (academic and nonacademic centers) in the United States and Canada.

Who Was Studied: Asymptomatic women presenting for screening mammography.

Who Was Excluded: Women who reported breast symptoms (e.g., lump, bloody or clear nipple discharge) at time of screening, had breast implants, reported possible pregnancy, had a mammogram within previous 11 months, or had a history of breast cancer treated with lumpectomy and radiation.

How Many Patients: 49,333 enrolled, 42,760 included in primary analysis

Study Overview: Multicenter randomized study. All women underwent both screen-film and digital mammography in random order. Digital and screen-film mammograms were interpreted independently by 2 radiologists, 1 reader for each examination. Mammograms were rated on a 7-point malignancy scale allowing for ROC analysis and BI-RADS classification. Diagnostic workup was performed if either reader recommended it.

Interventions: Participants were randomized to 1 of 2 treatment arms: (1) a 2-view screen-film mammogram followed by a 2-view digital mammogram of each breast; (2) a 2-view digital mammogram followed by a 2-view screen-film mammogram of each breast.

Follow-Up: Repeat screen-film or digital mammogram at 1 year, and a 455-day period after initial mammogram for any breast biopsy results.

Endpoints: Diagnostic accuracy of screen-film versus digital mammography, including sensitivity, specificity, positive predictive value, and areas under the curve (AUC).

RESULTS

- Digital and screen-film mammography had comparable diagnostic accuracy for the entire screening population with mean AUC of 0.78 ± 0.02 for digital and 0.74 ± 0.02 for screen-film mammography (difference, 0.03; 95% CI, −0.02 to 0.08; $P = 0.18$) (Table 40.1).
- Digital mammography was more accurate than screen-film mammography for women <50 years of age (AUC for digital mammography, 0.84 ± 0.03, AUC for screen-film, 0.69 ± 0.05; difference, 0.15; 95% CI, 0.05–0.25; $P = 0.002$), women with heterogeneously or extremely dense breasts (AUC for digital mammography, 0.78 ± 0.03, AUC for screen-film, 0.68 ± 0.03; difference, 0.11, 95% CI, 0.04–0.18; $P = 0.003$), and premenopausal or perimenopausal women (AUC for digital mammography, 0.82 ± 0.03, AUC for screen-film, 0.67 ± 0.05; difference, 0.15, 95% CI, 0.05–0.24; $P = 0.002$).

Table 40.1. THE TRIAL'S KEY FINDINGS

Performance Measure	Digital Mammography Value (± SD)	Screen-Film Mammography Value (± SD)	Difference P value[a]
All women			
Sensitivity	0.41 ± 0.03	0.41 ± 0.03	0.92
Specificity	0.98 ± 0.001	0.98 ± 0.001	0.006
PPV	0.12 ± 0.01	0.13 ± 0.01	
Women <50 years old			
Sensitivity	0.49 ± 0.06	0.35 ± 0.06	0.06
Specificity	0.97 ± 0.001	0.98 ± 0.001	0.07
PPV	0.08 ± 0.01	0.07 ± 0.01	
Women with dense breasts[b]			
Sensitivity	0.38 ± 0.04	0.36 ± 0.04	0.69
Specificity	0.97 ± 0.001	0.97 ± 0.001	0.33
PPV	0.10 ± 0.01	0.10 ± 0.01	
Premenopausal or perimenopausal women			
Sensitivity	0.47 ± 0.05	0.38 ± 0.05	0.20
Specificity	0.97 ± 0.001	0.98 ± 0.001	0.20
PPV	0.10 ± 0.01	0.09 ± 0.01	

SD = standard deviation; CI = confidence interval; PPV = positive predictive value.
[a] $P < 0.05$ is considered a statistically significant difference between groups.
[b] Includes women with heterogeneously dense or extremely dense breast tissue on mammography.

Criticisms and Limitations: DMIST did not determine mortality benefit of digital versus screen-film mammography. The 7-point malignancy scale used has not been validated in other large studies. The 455-day follow-up period is longer than the conventional 1-year follow-up period.

Other Relevant Studies and Information:

- Digital mammography offers additional advantages over screen-film mammography including improved transmission, retrieval, and storage of images, as well as lower average radiation dose.[2]
- An exploratory analysis of selected population subgroups in DMIST found that screen-film tended to perform better for women ≥65 years of age with fatty breasts, but nonsignificantly.[3]

- A quality-of-life substudy among DMIST participants surveyed shortly after screening and 1 year later found that false-positive mammograms were associated with increased transient short-term anxiety, and that there was no measurable health utility decrement.[4]
- Using discrete-event simulation modeling and DMIST data, digital mammography screening for all women was found to not be cost-effective relative to screen-film mammography, but age-targeted digital mammography screening is cost-effective.[5]
- Currently, the United States Preventive Services Task Force (USPSTF) recommends biennial mammography screening for women 50–74 years of age. The USPSTF recommends that the decision to start regular screening mammography before the age of 50 years be an individual one, taking into account the patient's values regarding specific benefits and harms. The USPSTF concluded that the current evidence is insufficient to make recommendations for women >74 years old.[6]
- The American Cancer Society and the American College of Radiology recommend annual screening mammography for women ≥40 years of age, and that they continue to do so for as long as they are in good health.[7,8]

Summary and Implications: Digital mammography has comparable diagnostic accuracy to screen-film mammography overall, but is more accurate than screen-film mammography among women <50 years of age, women with dense breasts, and premenopausal or perimenopausal women (Figure 40.1).

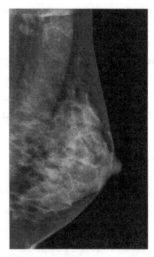

Figure 40.1 Normal digital MLO view mammogram of the left breast in a young woman with dense breast tissue. The craniocaudal (CC) view was equally unremarkable. No suspicious findings were identified.

CLINICAL CASE: DIGITAL OR SCREEN-FILM MAMMOGRAPHY?

Case History:

A 42-year-old female presents to your primary care clinic to discuss starting routine mammography screening after her best friend's recent breast cancer diagnosis. She is pre-menopausal and has no breast symptoms. While she understands the risks of false-positive screening exams, she is more interested in not missing a cancer and prefers to start mammography screening. She has no personal family history of breast cancer and has never had a breast biopsy. She asks which imaging modality is best and if such equipment is available within your health care system.

Suggested Answer:

Based on DMIST, digital mammography is more accurate than screen-film mammography for detecting cancers for women <50 years of age and pre-menopausal. Cancers detected by digital mammography and missed by screen-film mammography among these subgroups tend to be mostly invasive and high-grade ductal carcinoma in situ cases, suggesting that earlier detection may lead to improved outcomes. As >90% of all mammography units currently in use in the United States are now digital rather than screen-film, it is highly likely that digital mammography is available within her health care system.

References

1. Pisano ED, Gastonis C, Hendrick E, et al. Diagnostic performance of digital versus film mammography for breast-cancer screening. *N Engl J Med.* 2005;353(17):1773–1783.
2. Bloomquist AK, Yaffe MJ, Mawdsley GE, et al. Quality control for digital mammography in the ACRIN DMIST trial: part I. *Med Phys.* 2006;33(3):719–736.
3. Pisano ED, Hendrick RE, Yaffe MJ, et al. Diagnostic accuracy of digital versus film mammography: exploratory analysis of selected population subgroups in DMIST. *Radiology.* 2008;246(2):376–383.
4. Tosteson AN, Fryback DG, Hammond CS, et al. Consequences of false-positive screening mammograms. *JAMA Intern Med.* 2014;174(6):954–961.
5. Tosteson AN, Stout NK, Fryback DG, et al. Cost-effectiveness of digital mammography breast cancer screening. *Ann Intern Med* 2008;148(1):1–10.
6. US Preventive Services Task Force. Screening for breast cancer: U.S. Preventive Services Task Force recommendation statement. *Ann Intern Med* 2009;151(10):716–726.

7. American Cancer Society. American Cancer Society recommendations for early breast cancer detection in women without breast symptoms. http://www.cancer.org/cancer/breastcancer/moreinformation/breastcancerearlydetection/breast-cancer-early-detection-acs-recs. Accessed May 30, 2015.

8. Lee CH, Dershaw DD, Kopans D, et al. Breast cancer screening with imaging: recommendations from the Society of Breast Imaging and the ACR on the use of mammography, breast MRI, breast ultrasound, and other technologies for the detection of clinically occult breast cancer. *J Am Coll Radiol*. 2010;7(1):18–27.

41

Breast MRI for Women with Recently Diagnosed Breast Cancer

The American College of Radiology Imaging Network (ACRIN) Trial 6667

CHRISTOPH I. LEE

Our study shows that MRI can improve the detection of cancer in the contralateral breast when added to a thorough clinical breast examination and mammographic evaluation at the time of the initial diagnosis of breast cancer.

—LEHMAN ET AL.[1]

Research Question: Does MRI improve on clinical breast examination and mammography in detecting contralateral breast cancer in newly diagnosed breast cancer patients?

Funding: National Cancer Institute.

Year Study Began: 2003

Year Study Published: 2007

Study Location: 25 medical centers (academic and nonacademic) in the United States, Canada, and Germany.

Who Was Studied: Women ≥18 years of age with diagnosis of unilateral breast cancer within 60 days prior to the MRI, and negative or benign mammogram and clinical breast exam of the contralateral breast within the past 90 days.

Who Was Excluded: Previous breast MRI within 12 months before enrollment, pregnant, contraindication to MRI, breast cancer diagnosed >60 days prior to enrollment, or treated for breast cancer within 6 months before enrollment.

How Many Patients: 969

Study Overview: Multicenter, prospective cohort study with all eligible patients undergoing diagnostic breast MRI prior to definitive surgery. All breast MRI examinations were interpreted according to the American College of Radiology's Breast Imaging Reporting and Data System (BI-RADS). For purposes of receiver-operating-characteristics (ROC) curve analysis, MRI examinations were rated on a 5-point malignancy scale (1 "definitely not malignant" to 5 "definitely malignant). Cancer diagnosis (ductal carcinoma in situ [DCIS] and invasive) was based on histologic examination of biopsy samples.

Exposure: All patients underwent dynamic, contrast-enhanced breast MRI with minimum standard criteria (1.5-tesla or larger magnet, dedicated breast-surface coil).

Follow-Up: 365 days after breast MRI.

Endpoints: Primary endpoint was diagnostic yield of MRI for contralateral breast cancer. Secondary endpoints were sensitivity, specificity, negative predictive value, positive predictive value and associated positive biopsy rate, and estimation of the ROC curves for MRI.

RESULTS

- MRI detected contralateral breast cancer in 3.1% (30/969; 95% CI, 2.0%–4.2%) of patients that were clinically and mammographically occult (Table 41.1).
- MRI had a sensitivity of 91% (95% CI, 76%–98%), specificity of 88% (95% CI, 86%–90%), negative predictive value of 99% (95% CI, 99%–100%), and positive predictive value of a positive MRI examination of 21% (95% CI, 14%–27%).

- MRI led to a breast biopsy for a contralateral breast imaging finding in 12.5% of women (121/969), 24.8% (30/121) of whom had biopsies positive for cancer (18/30 were invasive cancer and 12/30 were DCIS; all node negative).
- The additional diagnostic yield of MRI was not influenced by breast density (fatty vs. dense), menopausal status (premenopausal or perimenopausal vs. postmenopausal), or tumor histologic features (invasive vs. in situ and lobular vs. nonlobular).
- The mean area under the ROC curve for MRI was 0.94 ± 0.02 (95% CI, 0.90–0.98) for the entire study cohort, and did not differ significantly between subgroups based on patient or tumor characteristics.
- The risk of occult cancer in the contralateral breast 1 year after a negative MRI was 0.3% (3/969); all 3 cancers detected were DCIS ≤4 mm in size.

Table 41.1. THE TRIAL'S KEY FINDINGS

Characteristic	Cancers Detected	Sensitivity	Specificity	NPV
All patients (n = 969)	3% (30/969)	91% (30/33)	88% (822/936)	99% (822/825)
Breast density				
Fatty	3% (9/299)	100% (9/9)	91% (264/290)	100% (264/264)
Dense	3% (20/666)	87% (20/23)	86% (555/643)	99% (555/558)
Menopausal status				
Pre/peri-	2% (8/414)	80% (8/10)	84% (339/404)	99% (339/341)
Postmenopausal	4% (22/552)	96% (22/23)	91% (480/529)	100% (480/481)
Tumor histology of index cancer				
Invasive ductal	63% (19/30)	95% (9/20)	88% (478/545)	100% (478/479)
Invasive lobular	20% (6/30)	100% (6/6)	87% (83/95)	100% (83/83)
DCIS	17% (5/30)	71% (5/7)	90% (170/189)	99% (170/172)

NPV = negative predictive value; DCIS = ductal carcinoma in situ.

Criticisms and Limitations: Not all patients underwent imaging and standard examination at 1-year follow-up, leaving the possibility of missed new cancers. The most appropriate follow-up period for calculating sensitivity, specificity, and negative and positive predictive values is unknown since lead-time distribution is unknown.

Other Relevant Studies and Information:

- Up to 10% of women have cancer found in the contralateral breast within 15 years of follow-up after receiving treatment for unilateral breast cancer despite normal findings on clinical and mammography examinations, thus requiring a second round of cancer therapy that could have been prevented if detected at time of initial diagnosis.[2,3]
- Compared to this trial's results, another study examining combined mammography and MRI screening in high-risk women showed an additional diagnostic yield from MRI of 1% and a sensitivity of 80%.[4]
- The NCCN suggests that breast MRI may be used for patients with a newly diagnosed breast cancer to evaluate the extent of ipsilateral disease and to screen the contralateral breast, particularly for women at increased risk for mammographically occult disease.[5]

Summary and Implications: Breast MRI in newly diagnosed unilateral breast cancer patients can detect contralateral early-stage breast cancers missed by mammography and clinical breast examination (Figure 41.1). In addition, breast MRI has an extremely high negative predictive value (99%), and may provide helpful information to women and physicians weighing the relative value of prophylactic contralateral mastectomy in the setting of unilateral breast cancer.

CLINICAL CASE: BREAST MRI IN NEWLY DIAGNOSED CANCER PATIENT

Case History:

A 42-year-old female presents to your breast surgery clinic with newly diagnosed left breast cancer. The patient felt a breast lump on her own about 3 months after her negative screening mammogram. On physical exam, she has a 2 cm mass in her upper outer quadrant of her left breast with some skin bruising from a recent ultrasound-guided biopsy. The right breast exam is unremarkable. By report, she has extremely dense breasts by mammography and no mammographic abnormalities bilaterally. She would like to discuss contralateral prophylactic mastectomy given the high tumor grade on histology. What would you recommend for this patient?

Suggested Answer:

Based on the ACRIN 6667 trial, this patient may benefit from the information provided by a diagnostic breast MRI. In this trial, 3.1% of patients newly diagnosed with unilateral breast cancer were found to have a contralateral early-stage breast cancer detected on MRI even in the setting of negative mammograms and clinical breast examination. Breast MRI also has a 99% negative predictive value, and would provide helpful information about disease status of the contralateral breast when weighing the risks and benefits of prophylactic contralateral mastectomy.

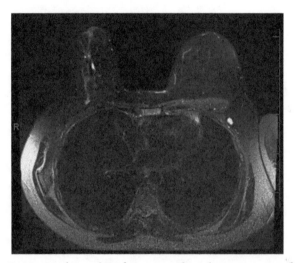

Figure 41.1 Contrast-enhanced T1 fat-saturated axial image as part of a right breast MRI-guided biopsy procedure. Note the small enhancing mass in the central right breast. This was found during MRI workup for the patient's newly diagnosed left-sided breast cancer.

References

1. Lehman CD, Gastsonis C, Kuhl CK, et al. MRI evaluation of the contralateral breast in women with recently diagnosed breast cancer. *N Engl J Med.* 2007;356(13):1295–1303.
2. Poggi MM, Danforth DN, Sciuto LC, et al. Eighteen-year results in the treatment of early breast carcinoma with mastectomy versus breast conservation therapy: the National Cancer Institute randomized trial. *Cancer.* 2003;98(4):697–702.
3. Veronesi U, Cascinelli N, Mariani L, et al. Twenty-year follow-up of a randomized study comparing breast-conserving surgery with radical mastectomy for early breast cancer. *N Engl J Med.* 2002;347(16):1227–1232.

4. Kriege M, Brekelmans CT, Boetes C, et al. Efficacy of MRI and mammography for breast-cancer screening in women with a familial or genetic predisposition. *N Engl J Med.* 2004;351(5):427–437.

5. Lehman CD, DeMartini W, Anderson BO, Edge SB. Indications for breast MRI in the patient with newly diagnosed breast cancer. *J Natl Compr Canc Netw.* 2009;7(2):193–201.

42

Supplemental Ultrasound Screening for Women at Increased Breast Cancer Risk

The ACRIN 6666 Trial

CHRISTOPH I. LEE

The addition of a single screening ultrasonographic examination to mammography for women at elevated risk of breast cancer results in increased detection of breast cancers that are predominantly small and node-negative.

—BERG ET AL.[1]

Research Question: Does adding screening ultrasound (US) to mammography for women at increased cancer risk detect additional cancers?

Funding: National Cancer Institute.

Year Study Began: 2004

Year Study Published: 2008

Study Location: 20 sites (academic and nonacademic) in the United States, Canada, and Argentina.

Who Was Studied: Women at elevated breast cancer risk, defined as having heterogeneously dense or extremely dense breast tissue in at least 1 quadrant and at least one other risk factor (personal history of breast cancer, lifetime risk ≥25% or 5-year risk ≥2.5% by Gail or Claus model, or 5-year risk ≥1.7% *and* known to have extremely dense breasts, prior atypical or lobular carcinoma in situ biopsy, *BRCA1* or *BRCA2* gene mutation, or prior radiation therapy to chest, mediastinum, or axilla prior to age 30 and at least 8 years earlier).

Who Was Excluded: Women with signs or symptoms of breast cancer; breast biopsy or procedure, MRI, or tomosynthesis within prior 12 months; mammography or whole breast ultrasound <11 months earlier; women with breast implants; pregnant, lactating, or planning to become pregnant within 2 years of study entry; known metastatic disease.

How Many Patients: 2,809

Study Overview: Prospective multicenter trial, randomized to the sequence of imaging modalities. Participants were randomized into 1 of 2 screening arms: (1) physician-performed bilateral handheld screening US followed by mammography within 2 weeks, or (2) mammogram followed by physician-performed bilateral screening US within 2 weeks. Imaging was performed using a standardized protocol, and radiologists used standardized criteria to interpret each examination while being masked to the other imaging results.

Exposures: Two-view mammography using either screen-film or digital mammography. Ultrasound performed with high-resolution linear array, broad bandwidth transducers with ≥12 MHz maximum frequency with color or power Doppler for noncystic lesions.

Follow-Up: Annually for 3 years.

Endpoints: Diagnostic cancer yield, sensitivity, specificity, diagnostic accuracy (area under the ROC curve), and positive predictive value (PPV) of biopsy recommendations for both screening strategies. The reference standard was a combination of pathology results within 365 days and clinical follow-up after 1 year.

RESULTS

- 40 women were diagnosed with cancer (39 with breast cancer), 8 detected by both US and mammography, 12 detected by US alone, 12 detected by mammography alone, and 8 not detected on either (Table 42.1).

- Of the 12 additional cancers detected by US alone, 92% (11/12) were invasive with a median size of 10 mm (range 5–40 mm, mean 12.6 mm) and 89% (8/9) were node-negative.
- The supplemental cancer yield after adding US screening (yield of 11.8/1,000 women) to mammography screening (yield 7.6/1,000 women) was 4.2 per 1,000 women screened (95% CI, 1.1–7.2/1,000).
- The diagnostic accuracy increased from 0.78 (95% CI, 0.67–0.87) to 0.91 (95% CI, 0.84–0.96) after adding supplemental US to mammography.
- The false-positive rate was 4.4% (95% CI, 3.7%–5.3%) for mammography alone, 8.1% (95% CI, 7.1%–9.2%) for ultrasound alone, and 10.4% (95% CI, 9.3%–11.7%) for mammography plus ultrasound, though this was incidence screening for mammography and prevalence screening for ultrasound.

Table 42.1. THE TRIAL'S KEY FINDINGS AT THE PARTICIPANT LEVEL

Screening Strategy	Cancer Detection Rate per 1,000[a]	Sensitivity[a]	Specificity[a]	PPV[a]
Mammography alone	7.6 (4.6–11.7)	50% (33.8%–66.2%)	95.5% (94.7%–96.3%)	14.7% (9.2%–21.8%)
Mammography plus ultrasound	11.8 (8–16.6)	77.5% (61.6%–89.2%)	89.4% (88.2%–90.6%)	10.1% (7.0%–14.1%)

Note: All performance characteristic differences between mammography alone and mammography plus ultrasound strategies were statistically significant ($P < 0.05$). PPV = positive predictive value of biopsy recommendation after full diagnostic workup.
[a]95% CI.

Criticisms and Limitations: For this trial, all ultrasounds were performed by subspecialty breast imaging radiologists; however, highly trained technologists using standard scanning techniques have been shown to approach similar performance measures.[2] The majority of patients had a personal history of breast cancer (n = 1,400, 53.09%), suggesting a high-risk population; thus, results may not be generalizable to women with dense breasts and no other risk factors (low- or intermediate-risk women). The median time to perform bilateral screening was 19 minutes, which may be problematic from the imaging workflow perspective.

Other Relevant Studies and Information:

- ACRIN 6666 findings corroborated previous reports that supplemental screening ultrasound can detect additional small, node-negative breast cancers not detected by mammography, with improved performance in women with dense breasts.[3-5]
- An Italian multicenter trial found that, among 6,449 women with dense breasts and negative mammogram results, 29 additional cancers were detected by screening US (cancer detection rate of 4.4/1,000).[6]
- In a follow-up analysis, the risk of false positives decreased significantly with annual combined mammography and ultrasound screening compared with the incident combined screening (PPV = 4.8% after first combined screen vs. 7.0% after subsequent combined screens) while still maintaining improved cancer detection (3.7 additional cancers per 1,000 women per year in both the second and third rounds, vs. 5.3 cancers per 1,000 women in the first round).[7]
- In the ACRIN 6666 follow-up analysis, with contrast-enhanced MRI within 8 weeks of final 24-month mammography and ultrasound screening round, MRI significantly increased detection of early breast cancer beyond that seen with combined mammography and ultrasound.[7] Screening MRI led to a supplemental cancer detection rate of 14.7 per 1,000 women, but at a high false-positive rate (PPV = 8.8%).
- Many states now have breast density reporting laws that require mammography facilities to directly inform women with dense breasts and negative screening mammography that they are at increased cancer risk and to discuss supplemental screening with their providers. Several of these states also mandate insurance coverage for supplemental ultrasound screening.[8]
- The American College of Radiology states that supplemental ultrasound screening "may be appropriate" for high-risk women (>20% lifetime risk, appropriateness score 6/9) and intermediate-risk women (15%–20% lifetime risk, appropriateness score 5/9, which includes women with dense breasts), but is "usually not appropriate" for average risk women (<15% lifetime risk, appropriateness score 2/9).[9]

Summary and Implications: Adding a single screening ultrasound to screening mammography for women at increased risk of breast cancer results in increased detection of cancers, mostly invasive and node-negative (Figure 42.1). The added detection of mostly invasive cancers comes at a substantial risk of false-positive results and benign biopsies in the first year that decrease moderately with incidence screening.

CLINICAL CASE: SUPPLEMENTAL SCREENING ULTRASOUND FOR WOMEN AT INCREASED BREAST CANCER RISK

Case History:

A 53-year-old female presents to your primary care clinic after receiving her mammography report in the mail. She was informed that she has dense breast tissue and should discuss potential supplemental screening with her physician. After a careful history, you learn that she had a mother who died of breast cancer at age 61, and she herself has had a previous benign breast biopsy. You determine that she is at intermediate risk (lifetime risk 15%–20%) of developing breast cancer using an available online risk assessment tool. How should you counsel this patient about supplemental ultrasound screening?

Suggested Answer:

Based on her intermediate risk status, there are both benefits and risks of supplemental ultrasound screening that this patient should consider. ACRIN 6666 demonstrated an increased detection of mammographically occult early invasive cancers, but with a risk of false-positive workups and benign biopsies. In addition, depending on your state, supplemental ultrasound may not be covered by the patient's insurance, and would require full payment out-of-pocket.

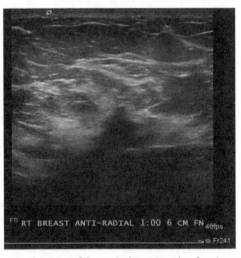

Figure 42.1 Ultrasound image of the right breast with a focal suspicious mass. The mass is hypoechoic, with angular/spiculated margins and posterior acoustic shadowing (all concerning characteristics for carcinoma).

References

1. Berg WA, Blume JD, Cormack JB, et al. Combined screening with ultrasound and mammography vs mammography alone in women at elevated risk of breast cancer. *JAMA*. 2008;299(18):2151–2163.

2. Berg WA, Mendelson EB. Technologist-performed handheld screening breast US imaging: how is it performed and what are the outcomes to date? *Radiology*. 2014;272(1):12–27.

3. Kolb TM, Lichy J, Newhouse JH. Comparison of the performance of screening mammography, physical examination, and breast US and evaluation of factors that influence them: an analysis of 27,825 patient evaluations. *Radiology*. 2002;225(1):165–175.

4. Buchberger W, Niehoff A, Obrist P, DeKoekkoek-Doll P, Dunser M. Clinically and mammographically occult breast lesions: detection and classification with high resolution sonography. *Semin Ultrasound CT MR*. 2000;21(4):325–336.

5. Crystal P, Strano SD, Shcharynski S, Koretz MJ. Using sonography to screen women with mammographically dense breasts. *AJR Am J Roentgenol*. 2003; 181(1):177–182.

6. Corsetti V, Ferrari A, Ghirardi M, et al. Role of ultrasonography in detecting mammographically occult breast carcinoma in women with dense breasts. *Radiol Med (Torino)*. 2006;111(3):440–448.

7. Berg WA, Zhang Z, Lehrer D, et al. Detection of breast cancer with addition of annual screening ultrasound or a single screening MRI to mammography in women with elevated breast cancer risk. *JAMA*. 2012;307(13):1394–1404.

8. DenseBreast-info.org. Legislation and regulations—what is required? http://densebreast-info.org/legislation.aspx. Revised February 26, 2016. Accessed August 28, 2015.

9. American College of Radiology. ACR appropriateness criteria: breast cancer screening. http://www.acr.org/~/media/ACR/Documents/AppCriteria/Diagnostic/BreastCancerScreening.pdf. Published 2012. Accessed June 2, 2015.

43

Chest Radiograph Screening for Lung Cancer

The Prostate, Lung, Colorectal, and Ovarian (PLCO) Cancer Screening Trial

CHRISTOPH I. LEE

> Annual screening with chest radiographs ... did not significantly decrease lung cancer mortality compared with usual care ...
>
> —OKEN ET AL.[1]

Research Question: Does annual screening with chest radiography lead to decreased lung cancer mortality?

Funding: National Cancer Institute.

Year Study Began: 1993

Year Study Published: 2011

Study Location: 10 screening centers: Georgetown University Medical Center, Henry Ford Health System, Marshfield Clinical Research Foundation, Pacific Health Research and Education Institute, University of Alabama at Birmingham, University of Colorado, University of Minnesota, University of Pittsburgh, University of Utah, and Washington University.

Who Was Studied: Men and women ages 55–74 years with no previous history of prostate, lung, colorectal, or ovarian (PLCO) cancer; unpaid volunteers recruited from the general population through mass mailings.

Who Was Excluded: Personal history of PLCO cancer; current cancer treatment; removal of 1 lung.

How Many Patients: 154,901

Study Overview: Randomized prospective multicenter trial. Patients were randomized to an intervention arm (organized screening program, n = 77,445) or control arm (usual care from health providers that sometimes included screening, n = 77,456), stratified by screening center, sex, and age.

Exposure: Intervention arm patients were offered annual single-view, posteroanterior (PA) chest radiograph for 4 years (only 3 years for never smokers randomized after 1995) (Figure 43.1). Diagnostic evaluation after a positive screening result (nodule, mass, infiltrate, or other abnormality) was left to the discretion of the patient's primary physician.

Follow-Up: Follow-up questionnaires by mail for up to 13 years from time of enrollment.

Endpoints: Primary endpoint was lung cancer mortality. Secondary outcomes included incidence of lung cancer, complications from diagnostic workup, and other-cause mortality.

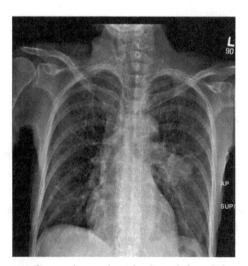

Figure 43.1 AP supine chest radiograph with a large left perhilar mass concerning for malignancy.

RESULTS

- In the intervention arm, screening adherence was 86.6% at baseline and decreased to 79% by year 3 (83.5% overall adherence rate). In the usual care arm, the contamination rate was 11% (control patients who underwent screening) (Table 43.1).
- Among 12,718 participants with at least 1 positive screen but no cancer eventually identified (false-positive screens), 15,445 had a diagnostic procedure, and 54 (0.4%) had a complication from the diagnostic workup (most common being pneumothorax, atelectasis, and infection).
- In the intervention group, 61% (307/505) of lung cancers were screen detected and 39% (198/505) were interval cancers. Screen-detected cancers were more likely to be adenocarcinoma (56%) and less likely to be small cell carcinoma (7%) compared to interval cancers. For non-small cell lung cancers, screened group cases were more likely to be stage I (32% vs. 27%) and less likely to stage IV (35% vs. 38%).
- After 13 years of follow-up, there were 1,213 lung cancer deaths in the intervention group and 1,230 in the usual care group (mortality rate ratio (RR): 0.99; 95% CI, 0.87–1.22). Both the lung cancer mortality RR and lung cancer incidence RR did not significantly differ by smoking history.
- Among a subset of participants eligible for the National Lung Screening Trial (NLST), the RR of lung cancer mortality was 0.94 (95% CI, 0.81–1.10) and the RR for lung cancer incidence was 1.00 (95% CI, 0.88–1.13).

Table 43.1. THE TRIAL'S KEY FINDINGS

Endpoint	Intervention Group (n = 77,445)	Usual Care Group (n = 77,456)	Rate Ratio (95% CI)
Lung cancer incidence (per 10,000 person-years)	20.1	19.2	1.05 (0.98–1.12)
Lung cancer mortality (per 10,000 person-years)	14.0	14.2	0.99 (0.87–1.22)
Other cause mortality (per 10,000 person-years)	11.7	11.9	0.98 (0.95–1.01)

Note: Rate ratios are the ratio of events between the intervention and usual care groups.

Criticisms and Limitations: Since the screening protocol only occurred the first 4 years, there is the possibility that the screening effect was diluted over time. Thus, both the absence of a mortality benefit and absence of a stage shift might have resulted, at least in part, due to the dilution effect.

Other Relevant Studies and Information:

- Previous smaller randomized trials, including the Mayo Lung Project and the Memorial Sloan-Kettering study, examining screening with sputum cytology and chest radiographs, did not detect lung cancer mortality reduction for the screening groups.[2,3]
- The NLST demonstrated a 20% lung cancer mortality reduction when higher-risk patients were screened with low-dose spiral CT rather than chest radiograph.[4]
- The American Lung Association no longer recommends screening for lung cancer using chest radiograph, and states that only low-dose spiral CT can reduce the risk of dying from lung cancer in high-risk populations.[5]
- The American Cancer Society and American College of Radiology, along with the USPSTF, recommends that annual screening with low-dose spiral chest CT be considered for apparently healthy patients at least 55 years of age who have at least a 30-pack-year smoking history and who currently smoke or have quit within the past 15 years.[6,7]

Summary and Implications: Annual chest radiograph screening over a 4-year period did not decrease lung cancer mortality compared with usual care after 13 years of follow-up. Chest x-rays are not an effective screening test for lung cancer.

CLINICAL CASE: CHEST RADIOGRAPH FOR LUNG CANCER SCREENING

Case History:
A 74 year-old male veteran presents to your clinic for hypertension medication management after recently transferring his care. Upon a full history and physical examination, you find that the patient is in relatively good health for his age, with moderate cardiovascular disease risk factors and a smoking history of 1 pack per day for 30 years. You ask him if he's been screened for lung cancer given his smoking history, and he states that his prior physician ordered annual chest radiographs for that purpose (Figure 43.1). He is interested in continuing screening. How would you counsel this patient?

Suggested Answer:
Based on the PLCO trial, there was no measurable mortality benefit from annual chest radiograph screening for lung cancer, regardless of smoking

history. You should begin with a discussion about the potential benefits versus risks of routine lung cancer screening, including the risks of false positives and unnecessary interventions with routine screening. If the patient chooses to undergo screening, he should not continue with chest radiographs but rather undergo low-dose spiral CT scans.

References

1. Oken MM, Hocking WG, Kvale PA, et al. Screening by chest radiograph and lung cancer mortality: the Prostate, Lung, Colorectal, and Ovarian (PLCO) randomized trial. *JAMA*. 2011;306(17):1865–1873.
2. Melamed MR, Flehinger BJ, Zaman MB, Heelan RT, Perchick WA, Martini N. Screening for early lung cancer: results of the Memorial Sloan-Kettering study in New York. *Chest*. 1984;86(1):44–53.
3. Fontana RS, Sanderson DR, Woolner LB, Taylor WF, Miller WE, Muhm JR. Lung cancer screening: the Mayo program. *J Occup Med*. 1986;28(8):746–750.
4. The National Lung Screening Trial Research Team. Reduced lung-cancer mortality with low-dose computed tomographic screening. *N Engl J Med*. 2011;365(5):395–409.
5. American Lung Association. Screening for lung cancer. http://www.lung.org/lung-disease/lung-cancer/learning-more-about-lung-cancer/diagnosing-lung-cancer/screening-for-lung-cancer.html. Accessed June 8, 2015.
6. Moyer VA; U.S. Preventive Services Task Force. Screening for lung cancer: U.S. Preventive Services Task Force recommendation statement. *Ann Intern Med*. 2014;160(5):330–338.
7. Wender R, Fontham ET, Barrera EJr, et al. American Cancer Society lung cancer screening guidelines. *CA Cancer J Clin*. 2013;63(2):107–117.

44

Low-Dose CT Screening for Lung Cancer

The National Lung Screening Trial (NLST)

CHRISTOPH I. LEE

> ... a 20.0% decrease in mortality from lung cancer was observed in the
> low-dose CT group as compared with the radiography group.
> —THE NLST RESEARCH TEAM.[1]

Research Question: Can annual low-dose CT screening for lung cancer among high-risk individuals decrease mortality?

Funding: National Cancer Institute.

Year Study Began: 2002

Year Study Published: 2011

Study Location: 33 US medical centers.

Who Was Studied: Participants were 55–74 years of age at the time of enrollment, had a history of cigarette smoking of at least 30 pack-years, and were either current smokers or quit within the previous 15 years.

Who Was Excluded: Individuals with previous lung cancer diagnosis, previous chest CT within 18 months of enrollment, hemoptysis, or unexplained weight loss (>15 lb) in the preceding year.

How Many Patients: 53,454

Study Overview: Multicenter randomized trial of screening with low-dose CT compared with chest radiography for lung cancer. Participants were randomly assigned to either 3 annual screening low-dose CT scans (n = 26,722) or single-view posteroanterior chest radiography (n = 26,732). Radiologists completed training in image quality and standardized image interpretation. Any noncalcified nodule or mass at least 4 mm in size were classified as positive and suspicious for lung cancer. At the third screening round, any suspicious abnormalities that were stable across the 3 rounds were classified as minor abnormalities rather than positive results.

Exposure: Standard protocols were used for all screening examinations. Low-dose CT scans were acquired with a minimum of a 4-channel multidetector CT scanner, with acquisition variables calibrated for an average effective dose of 1.5 mSv. Chest radiographs were obtained with either screen-film or digital equipment meeting American College of Radiology technical standards.

Follow-Up: Median follow-up of 6.5 years (maximum = 7.4 years) in each group. Follow-up included medical record abstraction for all diagnostic evaluations and complications after positive screening, annual or semiannual questionnaires, and search of National Death Index to ascertain vital status.

Endpoints: Primary endpoint was comparison of lung cancer mortality between the 2 screening groups using an intention-to-screen analysis. Secondary endpoints were all-cause mortality rate and lung cancer incidence in the two groups.

RESULTS

- Screening adherence rate was high across all three rounds for both the low-dose CT group (95%) and radiography group (93%) (Table 44.1).
- Across all 3 screening rounds, 39.1% in the low-dose CT group and 16.0% in the radiography group had at least 1 positive screening result. 96.4% of positive low-dose CT scans and 94.5% of positive radiographs were eventually determined to be false-positive results.
- 1,060 lung cancers were detected in the low-dose CT group (645/ 100,000 person-years) compared to 941 lung cancers in the radiography group (572 cases/100,000 person-years) (rate ratio, 1.13; 95% CI, 1.03–1.23).
- The lung cancer mortality rate with low-dose CT screening was 247 deaths per 100,000 person-years, compared with a rate of 309

deaths per 100,000 person-years in the radiography group, for a rate reduction of 20.0% ($P = 0.004$).

Table 44.1. THE TRIAL'S KEY FINDINGS

Outcome	Low-Dose CT Groupn	Radiography Groupn	Relative Rate Reduction[a]% (95% CI)
Lung cancer mortality	356	443	20.0% (6.8%–26.7%)
All-cause mortality	1,877	2,000	6.7% (1.2%–13.6%)

[a] Relative rate reduction is the reduction in mortality rate with low-dose CT screening compared to radiography screening.

Criticisms and Limitations: Since participants were enrolled on a volunteer basis, there may be a "healthy volunteer" effect. Newer-generation CT scanners may be more advanced and provide greater diagnostic accuracy compared to the scanners used in the NLST. The study took place in major medical centers, and community facilities may not be equipped to handle a lung cancer screening program. Since the comparator is chest radiography, low-dose CT effectiveness cannot be compared with usual care. Radiation-induced cancers and overdiagnosis are two potential risks of lung cancer screening that could not be directly addressed by the NLST.

Other Relevant Studies and Information:

- According to the Centers for Disease Control, approximately 7 million people in the United States would meet the eligibility criteria for the NLST.[2]
- The cost-effectiveness analysis of CT screening in the NLST demonstrated that low-dose CT screening would cost $81,000 per quality-adjusted life year (QALY) gained, meeting a cost-effectiveness threshold of $100,000 per QALY gained.[3] However, whether this approach is cost-effective in community settings will likely depend on the effectiveness of screening program implementation.
- A health-related quality of life study, which was part of the original trial, demonstrated that participants who received a false-positive or significant incidental finding result from screening experienced no significant anxiety or quality of life effects at 1 or at 6 months after screening relative to those who received a negative screening result.[4]
- An analysis using data from a subset of NLST participants found that smoking cessation was significantly associated with the identification

of screen-detected abnormalities. Thus, effective smoking cessation programs should be integrated into the screening program to further reduce morbidity and mortality.[5]

- The American Cancer Society and American College of Radiology, along with the USPSTF, recommend that annual screening with low-dose spiral chest CT be considered for apparently healthy patients at least 55 years of age who have at least a 30-pack-year smoking history and who currently smoke or have quite within the past 15 years.[6,7]

Summary and Implications: Annual low-dose CT screening among high-risk individuals decreases lung cancer mortality. While the rate of false positives is nearly 3 times higher for those screened by low-dose CT compared to chest radiography, complications from invasive diagnostic evaluation after positive screens are rare.

CLINICAL CASE: LOW-DOSE CT FOR LUNG CANCER SCREENING

Case History:
A 59-year-old female presents to your clinic wanting to discuss the possibility of going on a nicotine patch to quit smoking. She reports having been a smoker since her teenage years, at about a half pack a day. On physical exam and review of systems, she appears in relatively good health and denies hemoptysis, unexpected weight loss, or personal history of cancer. In addition to discussing smoking cessation programs, what other interventions could this patient potentially benefit from?

Suggested Answer:
This patient would meet the eligibility criteria of the NLST that showed a mortality reduction from annual low-dose spiral CT for lung cancer screening (Figure 44.1). The patient should be informed of both the benefits and risks of choosing to undergo routine CT screening, including the relatively high risk of a false-positive exam. The patient should also be informed that complications after diagnostic workup after positive screens are rare, and that any quality-of-life decrements from these additional workups appear to be transient. The patient should pursue an evidence-based smoking cessation program regardless of her choice to undergo or not undergo low-dose CT screening.

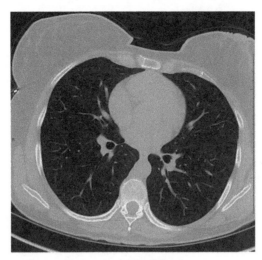

Figure 44.1 Normal noncontrast axial CT of the chest.

References

1. National Lung Screening Trial Research Team, Aberle DR, Adams AM, et al. Reduced lung-cancer mortality with low-dose computed tomographic screening. *N Engl J Med*. 2011;4(365):395–409.
2. Centers for Disease Control and Prevention. Cigarette smoking among adults and trends in smoking cessation—United States, 2008. *MMWR Morb Mortal Wkly Rep*. 2009;58(44):1227–1232.
3. Black WC, Gareen IF, Soneji SS, et al. Cost-effectiveness of CT screening in the National Lung Screening Trial. *N Engl J Med*. 2014;371(19):1793–1802.
4. Gareen IF, Duan F, Greco EM, et al. Impact of lung cancer screening results on participant health-related quality of life and state anxiety in the National Lung Screening Trial. *Cancer*. 2014;120(21):3401–3409.
5. Tammemägi MC, Berg CD, Riley TL, Cunningham CR, Taylor KL. Impact of lung cancer screening results on smoking cessation. *J Natl Cancer Inst*. 2014;106(6):dju0.84. doi:10.1093/jnci/dju084.
6. Moyer VA; US Preventive Services Task Force. Screening for lung cancer: U.S. Preventive Services Task Force recommendation statement. *Ann Intern Med*. 2014;160(5):330–338.
7. Wender R, Fontham ET, Barrera EJr, et al. American Cancer Society lung cancer screening guidelines. *CA Cancer J Clin*. 2013;63(2):107–117.

45

Management of Lung Nodules Detected by CT

CHRISTOPH I. LEE

> In a population that was at increased risk for lung cancer, our strategy of screening for lung cancer with the use of volume CT diminished the need for follow-up evaluation in participants with an indeterminate test result.
>
> —VAN KLAVEREN ET AL.[1]

Research Question: What is the best management strategy when noncalcified pulmonary nodules are incidentally identified on CT?

Funding: Zorg Onderzoek Nederland-Medische Wetenschappen, KWF Kankerbestrijding, Stichting Centraal Fonds Reserves van Voormalig Vrijwillige Ziekenfondsverzekeringen, G. Ph. Verhagen Foundation, Rotterdam Oncologic Thoracic Study Group, Erasmus Trust Fund, Foundation against Cancer, Flemish League against Cancer, Lokaal Gezondheids Overleg (LOGO) Leuven and Hageland, and Roche Diagnostics.

Year Study Began: 2003

Year Study Published: 2009

Study Location: Four medical centers in the Netherlands and Belgium.

Who Was Studied: Screened population of the Dutch-Belgian randomized lung cancer screening trial, also called the NELSON (Nederlands-Leuvens Longkanker Screenings Onderzoek) trial. Patients were born between 1928 and 1956 and were current or former smokers who quit smoking ≤10 years ago, smoked >15 cigarettes per day for >25 years, or >10 cigarettes per day for >30 years.

Who Was Excluded: Patients with moderate or bad self-reported health unable to climb 2 flights of stairs; body weight ≥ 140 kg; current or past renal cancer, melanoma, or breast cancer; lung cancer, diagnosed <5 years ago or ≥5 years ago but still under treatment; chest CT <1 year before enrollment.

How Many Patients: 7,557

Study Overview: Evaluation of a strategy using volume and volume-doubling time of noncalcified pulmonary nodules detected on CT to dictate an inexpensive diagnostic follow-up process without increasing the false-negative rate. Computer software was used to obtain semiautomated volume and volume growth measurements (LungCare software, Siemens Medical Solutions). Growth was defined as at least 25% volume change in between scans. Growing nodules were classified into three categories by volume-doubling time: <400, 400–600, and >600 days. Two radiologists independently interpreted the CT scan, with a third radiologist arbitrating any discrepant results. The workup, staging, and treatment were standardized across all screening sites based on published guidelines.

Exposure: Patients in the NELSON trial were randomly assigned to undergo no lung cancer screening or CT screening at baseline, 1 year, and 3 years later. CT scan protocols were standardized across sites, and were conducted on 16-detector CT scanners with images obtained in 1 mm thickness and reconstructed at overlapping 0.7 mm intervals. A screening test was considered negative if a nodule volume <50 mm^3, a nodule volume was 50–500 mm^3 but had not grown at 3-month follow-up CT, or if volume-doubling time was ≥400 days if it had grown at follow-up. If multiple nodules were present on a CT scan, then the largest volume or fastest growth determined the result.

Follow-Up: Two-year follow-up period.

Endpoints: Diagnostic sensitivity, specificity, positive predictive value, and negative predictive value at the participant level.

RESULTS

- After the first round of screening and short interval follow-up scans for indeterminate results, 97.4% (7,361/7,557) of participants had negative results and 2.6% (196/7,557) had positive results. The lung cancer detection rate was 0.9% (70/7,557), with 4 interval cancers not detected by screening (Table 45.1).
- After the second round of screening and short interval follow-up scans for indeterminate results, 98.2% (7,161/7,289) of participants had negative results and 1.8% (128/7,289) had positive results. The lung cancer detection rate was 0.5% (40/7,289) during the first year after second round of screening, and 0.8% (57/7,289) for the entire 2-year period after the second and third rounds of screening.
- Recall rates for CT scans among participants with indeterminate test results were 19.0% and 3.8% in screening rounds 1 and 2, respectively.
- Invasive diagnostic procedure rates were 1.2% and 0.8% in screening rounds 1 and 2, respectively.
- The chances for finding lung cancer on a CT scan at 3 months, 1 year, and 2 years after a negative baseline CT were 0, 1 in 1,000, and 3 in 1,000, respectively.

Table 45.1. THE TRIAL'S KEY FINDINGS

Round of Screening	Sensitivity % (95% CI)	Specificity % (95% CI)	PPV % (95% CI)	NPV % (95% CI)
First round	94.6% (86.5–98.0)	98.3% (98.0–98.6)	35.7% (29.3–42.7)	99.9% (99.9–100.0)
Second round	96.4% (86.8–99.1)	99.0% (98.7–99.2)	42.2% (33.9–50.9)	99.9% (99.9–100.0)

PPV = positive predictive value; NPV = negative predictive value; 95% CI = 95% confidence interval.

Criticisms and Limitations: The LungCare software did not automatically calculate volumetric data for all pulmonary nodules and had to be manually adjusted in 6.3% of detected nodules in the first round of screening, as well as 5.4% of new nodules and 1.9% of previously existing nodules in the second round of screening. Even though the software is not proprietary and can be used with any CT dataset, its use requires additional postprocessing manpower and interpretation time. The threshold values and ranges for volume-doubling time used were based on expert opinion and not definite, and could be improved. This strategy requires independent validation before its use can be widely adopted in lung cancer screening practices.

Other Relevant Studies and Information:

- The interval cancer rate and early (stage I) lung cancer detection rate found in the NELSON trial were similar to those found in other randomized trials.[2–4]
- Incidental pulmonary nodules are a common finding with the advent of multidetector CT, with some uncertainty about the best course of action among asymptomatic individuals at increased risk for lung cancer.[5]
- The American College of Chest Physicians recommends the following for individuals with a solid nodule and at least 1 risk factor for lung cancer[5]:
    1. Nodules ≤4 mm in diameter should be reevaluated at 12 months without the need for additional follow-up if unchanged.
    2. Nodules measuring >4 mm to 6 mm should be reevaluated sometime between 6–12 months and then again at 18–24 months if unchanged.
    3. Nodules measuring >6 mm to 8 mm should be initially reevaluated sometime between 3–6 months, then subsequently between 9–12 months, and again at 24 months if unchanged.

- The Fleischner Society has developed recommendation for follow-up and management of solid pulmonary nodules <8 mm in diameter incidentally detected at nonscreening CT for both patients without lung cancer risk factors and patients with lung cancer risk factors.[6] These recommendations are summarized in Table 45.2.

Summary and Implications: Volume-base measurements of pulmonary nodules may be an inexpensive and simple method for guiding the diagnostic follow-up process for indeterminate pulmonary nodules found on CT in high-risk individuals, without increasing the false-negative rate of CT lung cancer screening. The use of interval volume chest CT scans can lead to decreased need for invasive diagnostic evaluations without significant compromise to screening examination accuracy.

Table 45.2. FLEISCHNER SOCIETY RECOMMENDATIONS

Nodule Size (mm)	Low Risk for Lung Cancer	High Risk for Lung Cancer
≤4	No follow-up	Follow-up CT at 12 months; no further follow-up if unchanged
>4–6	Follow-up CT at 12 months; no further follow-up if unchanged	Follow-up CT at 6–12 months; at 18–24 months if unchanged
>6–8	Follow-up CT 6–12 months; at 18–24 months if unchanged	Follow-up CT at 3–6 months; at 9–12 months and 24 months if unchanged
>8	Follow-up CT at 3, 9, and 24 months; dynamic contrast-enhanced CT, PET, and/or biopsy	Follow-up CT at 3, 9, and 24 months; dynamic contrast-enhanced CT, PET, and/or biopsy

CLINICAL CASE: INDETERMINATE PULMONARY NODULE ON CT

Case History:

Your 56-year-old female patient underwent high-resolution CT for follow-up of bronchiectasis and small airway disease. Her chronic airway disease has improved with treatment; however, the thoracic radiologist found a new 5 mm solid pulmonary nodule in the lower lobe of the right lung (Figure 45.1). The patient has a 35-pack-year smoking history. What is your recommendation for follow-up CT, if any?

Suggested Answer:

This study from NELSON trial data suggests that interval CT scanning with volume measurements of small solid pulmonary nodules is an effective approach for management. Current society guidelines recommend an initial follow-up CT scan with volumetric measurements at 6–12 months for patients with at least 1 risk factor for lung cancer. If the size and volume of the pulmonary nodule has not changed at the initial follow-up CT scan, then another follow-up CT scan is recommended at 18–24 months. If unchanged at the second follow-up CT scan, no further follow-up is required. You should also discuss the potential benefits and risks of routine low-dose CT lung cancer screening with this patient with a significant smoking history.

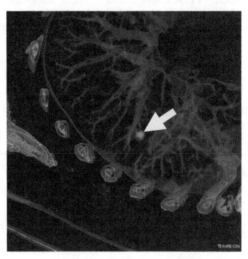

Figure 45.1 Volume-rendered and color-coded image of a right lower lobe lung nodule (arrow).

References

1. van Kleveren RJ, Oudkerk M, Prokop M, et al. Management of lung nodules detected by volume CT scanning. *N Engl J Med*. 2009;361(23):2221–2229.
2. Blanchon T, Bréchot JM, Grenier PA, et al. Baseline results of the Depiscan study: a French randomized pilot trial of lung cancer screening comparing low dose CT scan (LDCT) and chest X-ray (CXR). *Lung Cancer*. 2007;58(1):50–58.
3. Infante M, Lutman FR, Cavuto S, et al. Lung cancer screening with spiral CT: baseline results of the randomized DANTE trial. *Lung Cancer*. 2008;59(3):355–63.
4. Lopes Pegna A, Picozzi G, Mascalchi M, et al. Design, recruitment and baseline results of the ITALUNG trial for lung cancer screening with low-dose CT. *Lung Cancer*. 2009;64(1):34–40.
5. Gould MK, Donington J, Lynch WR, et al. Evaluation of individuals with pulmonary nodules: when is it lung cancer? Diagnosis and management of lung cancer, 3rd ed: American College of Chest Physicians evidence-based clinical practice guidelines. *Chest*. 2013;143(5 Suppl):e93S–e120S.
6. MacMahon H, Austin JH, Gamsu G, et al. Guidelines for management of small pulmonary nodules detected on CT scans: a statement from the Fleischner Society. *Radiology* 2005;237(2):395–400.

46

3D CT Colonography for Colorectal Cancer Screening

CHRISTOPH I. LEE

> Virtual colonoscopy not only had high sensitivity, but also maintained acceptable specificity for adenomas that were more than 6 mm in diameter ...
>
> —PICKHARDT ET AL.[1]

Research Question: How does 3D virtual colonoscopy (CT colonography) perform in an average-risk colorectal screening population?

Funding: Advanced in Medical Practice funds from the US Department of Defense.

Year Study Began: 2002

Year Study Published: 2003

Study Location: Three US medical centers.

Who Was Studied: Adults 50–79 years of age with an average risk of colorectal cancer and adults 40–79 years of age with a family history of colorectal cancer.

Who Was Excluded: Patients with positive stool guaiac test within previous 6 months; iron-deficiency anemia within previous 6 months; rectal bleeding or hematochezia within previous 12 months; unintentional weight loss (>10 lb) within previous 12 months; optical colonoscopy within previous 10 years; barium enema within previous 5 years; personal history of adenomatous polyp, colorectal cancer, or inflammatory bowel disease; family history for hereditary nonpolyposis cancer or familial adenomatous polyposis syndromes; inability to undergo optical colonoscopy; medical condition precluding sodium phosphate preparation; pregnancy.

How Many Patients: 1,233

Study Overview: Consecutively enrolled asymptomatic patients underwent same-day virtual and optical colonoscopy. Radiologists who received CT virtual colonoscopy interpretation training and had read a minimum of 25 virtual colonoscopy studies used 3D endoluminal display for initial detection of polyps. Experienced colonoscopists (14 gastroenterologists and 3 colorectal surgeons) were initially blinded to findings on virtual colonoscopy and used a standard commercial video colonoscope with a calibrated linear probe for photography of polyps. After the colonoscopist completed evaluation of a given segment of colon, a study coordinator revealed the results of the virtual colonoscopy for that previously examined segment, at which time the colonoscopist could reexamine the segment if a polyp >5 mm in diameter was detected on virtual colonoscopy but not on initial optical colonoscopy (including review of CT images for guidance). Time spent by patients for each procedure and time spent interpreting virtual colonoscopic studies were also recorded.

Exposure: Patients underwent standard 24-hour colonic preparation with oral sodium phosphate and bisacodyl, as well as oral contrast agents. Standardized CT protocol involved insertion of flexible rectal catheter and insufflation of room air into the colon immediately before scanning. Scans were performed with patient breath hold in both supine and prone positions, using a 4-channel or 8-channel CT scanner. 1.25- to 2.50-mm collimation was used with a 1 mm reconstruction interval. Postprocessing 3D images were created with a diagnostic interface allowing for a virtual "fly-through" tour of the images.

Follow-Up: Histologic evaluation of all polyps retrieved at optical colonoscopy. Medical record review for all extracolonic incidental findings.

Endpoints: Sensitivity and specificity of virtual colonoscopy and sensitivity of optical colonoscopy; reference standard was the finding of the final, unblinded optical colonoscopy.

RESULTS

- 97.4% (1,201/1,233) of study patients were at average risk. The other 2.6% (32/1,233) of patients had family histories that conferred a higher-than-average risk. The prevalence of adenomatous polyps did not significantly differ between patients with average risk and patients with higher-than-average risk.
- The sensitivity of virtual colonoscopy for all advanced neoplasms was 91.5% (54/59), while the sensitivity of optical colonoscopy for all advanced neoplasms was 88.1% (52/59) (Table 46.1).
- Two adenocarcinomas were detected among study patients, both detected by virtual colonoscopy, where 1 cancer (11 mm malignant polyp) was missed on optical colonoscopy before unblinding.
- 4.5% of patients (56/1,233) had extracolonic findings on CT of potentially high clinical importance. Unsuspected extracolonic cancer was ultimately found for 5 of these patients stemming from additional workup of these incidental findings (1 lymphoma, 2 bronchogenic carcinomas, 1 ovarian carcinoma, and 1 renal cell carcinoma). In addition, 2 patients underwent successful repair of unsuspected abdominal aortic aneurysms found incidentally on CT colonography.
- Patients spent a mean of 14.1 minutes in the CT suite versus 31.5 minutes in the endoscopy suite ($P < 0.001$). Mean time for optical colonoscopy increased to 95.9 minutes when including recovery after sedation. Mean time for interpretation of virtual colonoscopy studies was 19.6 minutes (median, 18.0 minutes).

Table 46.1. THE TRIAL'S KEY FINDINGS

Variable	Adenomatous Polyp Size Category % (no./total no.) [95% CI]		
	≥6 mm	≥8 mm	≥10 mm
Analysis according to patient			
Sensitivity of virtual colonoscopy	88.7% (149/168) [82.9–93.1]	93.9% (77/82) [86.3–98.0]	93.8% (45/48) [82.8–98.7]
Sensitivity of optical colonoscopy	92.3% (155/168) [87.1–95.8]	91.5%(75/82) [83.2–96.5]	87.5%(42/48) [74.8–95.3]
Analysis according to polyp			
Sensitivity of virtual colonoscopy	85.7%(180/210) [80.2–90.1]	92.6%(88/95) [85.4–97.0]	92.2%(47/51) [81.1–97.8]
Sensitivity of optical colonoscopy	90.0%(189/210) [85.1–93.7]	89.5%(85/95) [81.5–94.8]	88.2%(45/51) [76.1–95.6]

95% CI = 95% confidence interval.

Criticisms and Limitations: The optical colonoscopy was used as a gold standard in this study, but prior reports suggest that 6% of adenomas ≥10 mm in size are missed on back-to-back colonoscopies.[2] Patients with a suspicious polyp detected by virtual colonoscopy would still have to undergo optical colonoscopy in order to resect the polyp and obtain a histopathologic diagnosis. Incidental extracolonic findings on CT for average-risk adults require additional diagnostic studies and are not uncommon, but are less than half that reported in higher-risk populations.[3]

Other Relevant Studies and Information:

- Trials of virtual colonoscopy primarily using a 2D approach to interpretation among symptomatic and/or higher-risk individuals showed an average sensitivity for detecting polyps ≥10 mm in size of only 48%–55%.[4,5]
- The primary target of screening is adenomas (particularly advanced lesions) at least 6 mm in diameter. Consensus is that small colonic polyps <5 mm in size should be regarded as clinically insignificant and ignored on virtual colonoscopy.[6]
- The American Cancer Society, the US Task Force on Colorectal Cancer, and the American College of Radiology joint guidelines list multiple options as acceptable choices for colorectal cancer screening. These include CT colonography every 5 years, flexible sigmoidoscopy every 5 years, colonoscopy every 10 years, or double contrast barium enema every 5 years.[7]
- The American College of Gastroenterology recommends colon cancer screening starting at age 50, with colonoscopy every 10 years the preferred screening strategy. For patients declining or those ineligible for colonoscopic evaluation, CT colonography every 5 years should be offered as a potential alternative.[8]
- In their 2008 recommendations, the USPSTF concluded that there was insufficient evidence to assess the benefits and harms of CT colonography as a screening modality for colorectal cancer.[9]

Summary and Implications: Virtual colonoscopy, using a primary 3D approach for polyp detection, represents a minimally invasive procedure that is an accurate method for screening average-risk individuals. The likelihood of a clinically significant adenoma being missed on virtual colonoscopy is extremely low given the high negative predictive values.

CLINICAL CASE: VIRTUAL VERSUS OPTICAL COLONOSCOPY

Case History:

A 60-year-old male in good health presents to your primary care clinic for a routine preventive medicine checkup. He recently heard that President Obama had chosen to undergo virtual colonoscopy rather than traditional colonoscopy for colorectal cancer screening, and wanted to know if this could be an option for him. How would you counsel this patient?

Suggested Answer:

This study demonstrated that CT colonography (virtual colonoscopy) is a relatively accurate method for detecting large polyps in average-risk individuals, especially with a primary 3D interpretation method (Figure 46.1). There are mixed recommendations among experts regarding whether CT colonography can be used as a primary screening tool, or only as an alternative to optical colonoscopy for patients that are not eligible or decline optical colonoscopy. Most major societies agree that early detection and screening of any kind for colorectal cancer is the overall goal, and if this patient declines optical colonoscopy, CT colonography should be offered as an acceptable option.

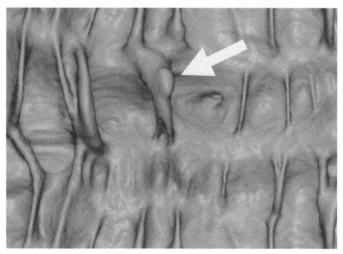

Figure 46.1 CT colonography 3D volume rendered image of a small colon polyp (arrow).

References

1. Pickhardt PJ, Choi JR, Hwang I, et al. Computed tomographic virtual colonoscopy to screen for colorectal neoplasia in asymptomatic adults. *N Engl J Med.* 2003;349(23):2191–2200.
2. Rex DK, Culter CS, Lemmel GT, et al. Colonoscopic miss rates of adenomas determined by back-to-back colonoscopies. *Gastroenterology.* 1997;112(1):24–28.
3. Gleucker TM, Johnson CD, Wilson LA, et al. Extracolonic findings at CT colonography: evaluation of prevalence and cost in a screening population. *Gastroenterology.* 2003;124(4):911–916.
4. Johnson CD, Harmsen WS, Wilson LA, et al. Prospective blinded evaluation of computed tomographic colonography for screen detection of colorectal polyps. *Gastroenterology.* 2003;125(2):311–319.
5. Durkalski VL, Palesch YY, Pineau BC, Vining DJ, Cotton PB. The virtual colonoscopy study: a large multicenter clinical trial designed to compare two diagnostic screening procedures. *Control Clin Trials.* 2002;23(5):570–583.
6. Winawer SJ, Zauber AG. The advanced adenoma as the primary target of screening. *Gastrointest Endosc Clin N Am.* 2002;12(1):1–9.
7. Levin B, Lieberman DA, McFarland B, et al. Screening and surveillance for the early detection of colorectal cancer and adenomatous polyps, 2008: a joint guideline from the American Cancer Society, the US Multi-Society Task Force on Colorectal Cancer, and the American College of Radiology. *CA Cancer J Clin.* 2008;58(3):130–160.
8. Rex DK, Johnson DA, Anderson JC, et al. American College of Gastroenterology guidelines for colorectal cancer screening 2009. *Am J Gastroenterol.* 2009;104(3):739–750.
9. US Preventive Services Task Force. Screening for colorectal cancer: U.S. Preventive Services Task Force recommendation statement. *Ann Intern Med.* 2008;149(9):627–637.

47

National CT Colonography Trial

The ACRIN 6664 Trial

CHRISTOPH I. LEE

> The less invasive nature of CT colonography and the low risk of procedure-related complications, as compared with colonoscopy, may be attractive to patients and may improve screening-adherence rates . . .
> —JOHNSON ET AL.[1]

Research Question: What is the accuracy of multidetector CT colonography for detecting large adenomas and cancers?

Funding: National Cancer Institute.

Year Study Began: 2005

Year Study Published: 2008

Study Location: 15 US medical centers (academic and nonacademic).

Who Was Studied: Adult patients ≥50 years old scheduled for screening colonoscopy.

Who Was Excluded: Patients with lower gastrointestinal tract disease symptoms (melena and/or hematochezia on more than one occasion in previous

6 months, lower abdominal pain requiring medical evaluation); inflammatory bowel disease and/or familial polyposis syndrome; serious medical conditions making screening difficult or of little benefit; pregnancy; previous colonoscopy within 5 years; anemia; positive fecal occult blood test.

How Many Patients: 2,600 enrolled, 2,531 with CT colonographic and colonoscopic results

Study Overview: Multicenter efficacy study. Radiologists trained in CT colonography reported all polyps ≥5 mm in size. Study data were randomly assigned to be read independently with either a primary 2D search method (with 3D endoluminal problem-solving), or a primary 3D search method (with capability of displaying multiplanar 2D images). Optical colonoscopy and histologic review served as the reference standard. A positive result on CT colonography was defined as identification of a lesion measuring ≥5 mm in size.

Exposure: CT was acquired with standard bowel preparation, stool and fluid tagging, mechanical insufflation, and multidetector-row CT scanners (16 or more rows) (Figure 47.1). Images were acquired with patients in supine and prone positions, and reconstructed to slice thickness of 1.0–1.25 mm, with a reconstruction interval of 0.8 mm. Index colonoscopy was performed by an experienced gastroenterologist or surgeon without knowledge of the CT colonographic results.

Follow-Up: 4-week follow-up.

Endpoints: Sensitivity, specificity, area under the ROC curve, and predictive values of CT colonography versus colonoscopy with regard to detecting large adenomas and adenocarcinomas (≥10 mm).

RESULTS

- A total of 128 large adenomas or carcinomas were found among 4% (109/2,531) of patients. If all patients with lesions ≥5 mm were referred to colonoscopy, the referral rate would be 17%. If all patients with lesions ≥6 mm were referred to colonoscopy, the referral rate would be 12% (Table 47.1).
- Pooled sensitivities for detecting large lesions using a primary 2D conventional software versus a primary 3D endoluminal fly-through software were not significantly different: 0.87 (95% CI, 0.75–0.95) and 0.88 (95% CI, 0.76–0.95), respectively.

- 66% of participants had extracolonic incidental findings on CT, but only 16% were considered significant and requiring additional evaluation.

Table 47.1. THE TRIAL'S KEY FINDINGS

Performance Measure[a]	Size of Adenoma/Cancer on Colonoscopy value (95% CI)		
	≥6 mm	≥8 mm	≥10 mm
Sensitivity	0.78 (0.71–0.85)	0.87 (0.80–0.93)	0.90 (0.84–0.96)
Specificity	0.88 (0.84–0.92)	0.87 (0.83–0.91)	0.86 (0.81–0.90)
Positive predictive value	0.40 (0.34–0.46)	0.31 (0.26–0.36)	0.23 (0.19–0.27)
Negative predictive value	0.98 (0.97–0.98)	0.99 (0.98–0.99)	0.99 (0.99–1.00)
Area under ROC curve	0.84 (0.81–0.88)	0.88 (0.84–0.91)	0.89 (0.85–0.93)

[a] Estimated per-patient accuracy of CT colonography for detecting adenoma or carcinoma.
ROC = receiver operating characteristic. 95% CI = 95% confidence interval.

Criticisms and Limitations: Participating radiologists were trained and experienced interpreters of CT colonography, so sensitivity among general radiologists in community settings may be lower. Since colonoscopy is not a perfect test but was used as the reference standard, reported CT colonography performance measures may be underestimated.

Other Relevant Studies and Information:

- While the higher accuracy seen by Pickhardt et al. compared to other studies was attributed to a primary 3D endoluminal reading technique,[2] this study showed similar performance between 2D and 3D primary image-display methods.
- One controversial study suggests that, including follow-up CT scans for extracolonic incidental findings, CT colonography is associated with a 0.15% increased risk of radiation-induced cancer for an individual undergoing screening every 5 years from age 50 until age 80.[3]
- The American Cancer Society, the US Task Force on Colorectal Cancer, and the American College of Radiology joint guidelines list multiple options as acceptable choices for colorectal cancer screening.

These include CT colonography every 5 years, flexible sigmoidoscopy every 5 years, colonoscopy every 10 years, or double contrast barium enema every 5 years.[4]

- The American College of Gastroenterology recommends colon cancer screening starting at age 50, with colonoscopy every 10 years the preferred screening strategy. For patients declining or those ineligible for colonoscopic evaluation, CT colonography every 5 years should be offered as a potential alternative.[5]
- In their 2008 recommendations, the USPSTF concluded that there was insufficient evidence to assess the benefits and harms of CT colonography as a screening modality for colorectal cancer.[6]

Summary and Implications: In this trial, CT colonography identified 90% of participants with adenomas or cancers measuring ≥10 mm. Results provide more evidence for CT colonography as an effective screening tool among asymptomatic average-risk individuals, but CT colonography does have lower sensitivity for smaller colorectal lesions (6–9 mm).

CLINICAL CASE: BENEFITS AND RISKS OF CT COLONOGRAPHY

Case History:

A 64-year-old female of average risk for colorectal cancer is trying to decide between traditional and CT colonography. She has investigated much of the literature via the Internet, and would like your opinion regarding the risks and benefits of the two tests before she makes her decision. What are the major benefits and risks that should be outlined?

Suggested Answer:

The ACRIN 6664 Trial showed that CT colonography identified 90% of participants with large polyps (≥10 mm). However, these results would indicate up to 1 in 10 participants undergoing CT colonography may have a large polyp missed. Thus, most major societies recommend that CT colonography be performed every 5 years, whereas optical colonoscopy need only be performed every 10 years. Both procedures require complete bowel preparation. The major risks of optical colonoscopy are related to polypectomy complications, with rare but potentially serious risks from perforation and bleeding. For CT colonography, the patient should be informed that any polyp ≥6 mm in size detected by CT will require an optical colonoscopy for further investigation. Minor risks include radiation exposure and the discovery of incidental extracolonic findings possibly requiring additional diagnostic workup.

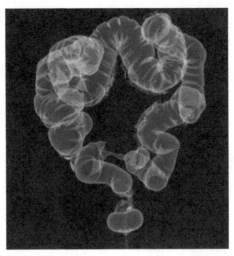

Figure 47.1 CT colonography 3D surface rendered image of the entire course of the colon.

References

1. Johnson CD, Chen M, Toledano AY, et al. Accuracy of CT colonography for detection of large adenomas and cancers. *N Engl J Med*. 2008;359(12):1207–1217.
2. Pickhardt PJ, Choi JR, Hwang I, et al. Computed tomographic virtual colonoscopy to screen for colorectal neoplasia in asymptomatic adults. *N Engl J Med*. 2003;349(23):2191–2200.
3. Berrington de González A, Kim KP, Knudsen AB, et al. Radiation-related cancer risks from CT colonography screening: a risk-benefit analysis. *AJR Am J Roentgenol*. 2011;196(4):816–823.
4. Levin B, Lieberman DA, McFarland B, et al. Screening and surveillance for the early detection of colorectal cancer and adenomatous polyps, 2008: a joint guideline from the American Cancer Society, the US Multi-Society Task Force on Colorectal Cancer, and the American College of Radiology. *CA Cancer J Clin*. 2008;58(3):130–160.
5. Rex DK, Johnson DA, Anderson JC, et al. American College of Gastroenterology guidelines for colorectal cancer screening 2009. *Am J Gastroenterol*. 2009;104(3):739–750.
6. US Preventive Services Task Force. Screening for colorectal cancer: U.S. Preventive Services Task Force recommendation statement. *Ann Intern Med*. 2008;149(9):627–637.

Radiation Exposure

48

Cancer Risk from Pediatric CT

CHRISTOPH I. LEE

> We hope that pointing out that lifetime radiation risks for children undergoing CT are quantitatively not negligible will encourage more active reduction of CT exposure settings in the pediatric context.
>
> —BRENNER ET AL.[1]

Research Question: What are the lifetime cancer mortality risks attributable to radiation from pediatric CT?

Funding: United States Department of Energy, National Cancer Institute.

Year Study Published: 2001

Study Overview: Lifetime cancer mortality risks per unit dose as a function of age at exposure were obtained from the National Academy of Sciences Biological Effects of Ionizing Radiation committee and the International Commission on Radiological Protection.[2,3] Doses for pediatric CT examinations were estimated from a 1989 survey of CT practice in Britain in which adult organ doses were estimated for 17 types of CT examinations from >100 CT scanners.[4,5] Age-dependent lifetime cancer mortality risks per unit dose were then multiplied with estimated age-dependent doses produced by various CT examinations.

Endpoints: Estimates of lifetime age-dependent cancer mortality risks associated with two of the most common CT examinations among pediatric patients—head CT and abdominal CT.

RESULTS

- Total number of deaths attributable to 1 year (2001) of CT examinations in the U.S. is approximately 700 from head CTs and 1,800 from abdominal CT examinations in patients <15 years old.
- Estimated lifetime cancer mortality risks attributable to radiation exposure in a 1-year-old are approximately 1 in 550 (0.18%) for an abdominal CT and 1 in 1,500 (0.07%) for a head CT. These estimates are an order of magnitude higher than risks for adults.
- If 600,000 abdominal and head CTs are performed annually among pediatric patients <15 years of age, then roughly 500 may eventually die from radiation-induced cancer.

- Estimated lifetime cancer mortality risks from abdominal CT examinations are greater for female patients than for male patients due to significantly greater risks per unit dose for digestive organ cancer in women.

Criticisms and Limitations: Data on radiation-induced cancer per unit dose inherently assume a linear extrapolation of risks for low-dose radiation from intermediate-dose radiation (linear no-threshold model, with risk estimates derived from mortality data of Japanese atomic bomb survivors). Relative effective doses for children were scaled from estimated organ doses for adult CT examinations. This analysis assumed that pediatric CT examinations used the same milliampere-second (mA-s) techniques of adult CT examinations. While absolute estimated risks were high, the percentage increase in cancer mortality beyond natural background rates was very low.

Other Relevant Studies and Information:

- Relative risk mechanism for radiation-induced cancer purports that the lifetime risk attributable to a single small dose of radiation is larger for children than adults (who face a larger lifetime background risk of cancer mortality).

- Since this study was published, the Alliance for Radiation in Pediatric Imaging has promoted the Image Gently campaign to decrease radiation exposure among pediatric patients worldwide.[6]
- The American College of Radiology and the Radiological Society of North America have promoted the Image Wisely campaign to ensure that all patients undergo imaging only when clinically indicated and that they receive doses as low as reasonably achievable.[7]
- From 1995 to 2008, pediatric CT use in the US emergency department setting increased from 0.33 million to 1.65 million, with an annual growth rate of 13.2%.[8]

Summary and Implications: Pediatric patients are at significantly increased lifetime radiation risks from CT compared to adults. Every effort should be made to eliminate unnecessary radiation exposure among pediatric patients, and to lower the mA-s and increase pitch settings of CT for children, without significant loss of clinically relevant information.

CLINICAL CASE: RADIATION RISKS FROM PEDIATRIC CT

Case History:
A 9-year-old boy arrives in the emergency department with lower abdominal pain. The patient has a low-grade fever and elevated white blood cell count. Targeted right lower quadrant ultrasound did not identify the appendix. Before ordering an abdominal CT scan to evaluate for suspected appendicitis, what type of information should you provide the parents during the informed consent process, and what should you ensure in terms of the examination itself?

Suggested Answer:
In a pediatric patient with suspected acute disease, such as appendicitis, the benefits of CT scan far outweigh the small lifetime attributable cancer risks. Nevertheless, radiation-induced cancer is a potential risk and should be listed along with contrast reaction as a potential harm during the informed consent process. Larson et al found that parents' willingness to have their children undergo CT recommended by their doctor did not change after being informed of potential future radiation-induced cancer risks.[9] For the examination itself, pediatric dose settings or low-dose techniques should be implemented to keep doses as low as reasonably achievable.

References

1. Brenner DJ, Elliston CD, Hall EJ, Berdon WE. Estimated risks of radiation-induced fatal cancer from pediatric CT. *AJR Am J Roentgenol.* 2001;176(2):289–296.
2. BEIR V (Committee on the Biological Effects of Ionizing Radiations). *Health effects of exposure to low levels of ionizing radiation.* Washington, DC: National Academies Press; 1990.
3. International Commission on Radiological Protection. 1990 recommendations of the International Commission on Radiological Protection. ICRP Publication 60. *Ann ICRP.* 1991:21(1–3).
4. Shrimpton PC, Jones DG, Hillier MC, Wall BF, Le Heron JC, Faulkner K. *Survey of CT practice in the UK. 2. Dosimetric aspects. NRPB Report 249.* Chilton, England: National Radiological Protection Board; 1991.
5. Huda W, Atherton JV, Ware DE, Cumming WA. An approach for the estimation of effective radiation dose at CT in pediatric patients. *Radiology.* 1997;203(2):417–422.
6. Alliance for Radiation in Pediatric Imaging. Image Gently. http://www.image-gently.org. Accessed August 2, 2015.
7. Brink JA, Amis ES Jr. Image Wisely: a campaign to increase awareness about adult radiation protection. *Radiology.* 2010;257(3):601–602.
8. Larson DB, Johnson LW, Schnell BM, Goske MJ, Salisbury SR, Forman HP. Rising use of CT in child visits to the emergency department in the United States, 1995–2008. *Radiology.* 2011;259(3):793–801.
9. Larson DB, Rader SB, Forman HP, Fenton LZ. Informing parents about CT radiation exposure in children: it's OK to tell them. *AJR Am J Roentgenol.* 2007;189(2):271–275.

49

Imaging Utilization Trends and Radiation Exposure

CHRISTOPH I. LEE

> Within integrated health care systems, there was a large increase in the rate of advanced diagnostic imaging and associated radiation exposure between 1996 and 2010.
> —SMITH-BINDMAN ET AL.[1]

Research Question: What are the trends in imaging utilization and associated radiation exposure among members of integrated health care systems?

Funding: National Cancer Institute.

Year Study Began: Data from 1996 through 2010

Year Study Published: 2012

Study Location: Six geographically diverse, large, integrated US health systems (all members of the HMO Research Network).

Who Was Studied: Member-patients of integrated health care systems that have both care delivery and insurance relationships with their members. Included were all members enrolled in group- and staff-model plans, commercial plans, Medicaid, and Medicare Advantage plans.

Who Was Excluded: Health plan members with fee-for-service (network) plans and patients treated at health plan facilities without being enrolled in the HMO plans.

How Many Patients: Between 933,897 and 1,998,650 patients annually from 1996 to 2010.

Study Overview: Retrospective analysis of electronic records of members from 6 health systems. The Virtual Data Warehouse, a data resource utility, was used to capture standardized imaging data from electronic medical and administrative records. Effective dose for each CT examination was estimated using parameters extracted from the Digital Imaging and Communications in Medicine tags stored in the Picture Archiving and Communications Systems for a random selection of patients undergoing CT based on age and sex each year from across the participating sites. These parameters included the body region, scan length, kilovolt peak, milliamperes or mA-seconds, rotation time, pitch, and CT machine model. Effective doses for examinations of other imaging modalities were derived from various published and unpublished estimates.

Study Intervention: All diagnostic imaging tests were included (radiation therapy–related imaging was excluded). A total of 1,467 unique imaging ICD-9 codes were captured across all years, with 1,068 of them associated with ionizing radiation.

Endpoints: Advanced diagnostic imaging utilization rates (number of imaging examinations/1,000 enrollees per year) and cumulative annual radiation exposure from medical imaging (per capita dose in mSv/person/year).

RESULTS

- During the 15-year study period, enrollees underwent a total of 30.9 million imaging examinations, or an average of 1.18 imaging examinations per person per year (95% CI, 1.17–1.19).
- While utilization of radiography and angiography remained relatively stable over time, utilization of advanced imaging changed markedly over time (Table 49.1).
- During the study period, computed tomography utilization experienced a 7.8% annual growth rate (95% CI, 5.8%–9.8%), magnetic resonance imaging utilization experienced a 10% annual growth rate (95% CI, 3.3%–16.5%), and ultrasound experienced a 3.9% annual growth rate (95% CI, 3.0%–4.9%).

- While nuclear medicine utilization rates decreased over time, the use of PET imaging experienced a 57% annual growth rate (0.24/1,000 enrollees in 1996 to 3.6/1,000 enrollees in 2010).
- Mean per capita effective dose from medical imaging increased from 1.2 mSv in 1996 to 2.3 mSv in 2010, mostly from the increased utilization of computed tomography.
- For individuals who were exposed to any radiation from medical imaging, the average effective dose increased from 4.8 mSv in 1996 to 7.8 mSv in 2010 (3.2% annual growth rate; 95% CI, 3.1%–3.3%).
- By 2010, 10.8% of member-patients received an annual effective dose >20 mSv, suggesting more intensive imaging among a subset of patients undergoing any imaging.

Table 49.1. THE STUDY'S KEY FINDINGS

Imaging Modality	Examination Rates per 1,000 Enrollees (Average per Capita Radiation Dose, mSv)		
	1996	2003	2010
Computed Tomography	52 (0.38)	108 (0.90)	149 (1.58)
Nuclear Medicine	32 (0.17)	45 (0.26)	21 (0.19)
Angiography/Fluoroscopy	68 (0.52)	64 (0.49)	57 (0.34)
Radiography	610 (0.17)	668 (0.21)	722 (0.22)
Magnetic Resonance[a]	17	41	65
Ultrasound[a]	134	186	230

mSv = millisieverts.

[a] Magnetic resonance imaging and ultrasound do not impart ionizing radiation; thus, no average per capita radiation doses are provided.

Criticisms and Limitations: Fee-for-service enrollees were excluded from the analysis due to incomplete data. Patients who underwent multiple examinations with the same procedure code on the same day were only counted once, underestimating their exposure. Dose estimates were used rather than actual dose information for each examination.

Other Relevant Studies and Information:

- Effective dose quantifies the probability of cancer induction and genetic effects of ionizing radiation, taking into account the nature of each organ or tissue that is irradiated. It is, therefore, a measure of overall detrimental biological effect of a radiation exposure.
- For context regarding levels of patient radiation exposure, governmental limits on occupational radiation exposure are 20 mSv

annually in Europe and 50 mSv annually in the United States.[2,3] In addition, a dose of 10 mSv is believed to put an individual at increased risk of developing cancer.[4] In this study, by 2010, 10.8% of enrollees who underwent imaging received an annual exposure >20 mSv.

- Increasing utilization rates of advanced imaging are similar between HMO and Medicare fee-for-service insured beneficiaries. Rates of computed tomography imaging increased an average of 10.2% annually between 1998 and 2005 for HMO enrollees ≥65 years, compared to 10.1% among Medicare fee-for-service beneficiaries for the same time period.[5]

Summary and Implications: Similar to the fee-for-service insured population, the utilization rates for advanced imaging in the integrated health system population increased substantially from 1995 to 2010. Given the potential radiation-induced cancer risks associated with advanced imaging, the clinical benefits of advanced imaging should be quantified to determine the relative risk-benefit ratios of advanced imaging procedures.

CLINICAL CASE: IMAGING UTILIZATION TRENDS

Case History:
Your institution, an integrated healthcare system, would like to curb inappropriate use of advanced imaging, including CT, MRI, and nuclear medicine imaging examinations. Since radiology benefits managers cannot be used in this setting to control imaging utilization and costs (as they are in private commercial payer settings), the leadership has come to you as the quality improvement expert to help institute a computerized decision support system. What is the current evidence regarding computer physician order entry with decision support for advanced imaging utilization?

Suggested Answer:
While early, single-institution studies suggested a significant decrease in advanced imaging utilization after instituting computer physician order entry with decision support software, a recent Centers for Medicare and Medicaid Services Demonstration Project showed that such systems did not significantly curb inappropriate advanced imaging utilization.[6] One limitation cited was the heavy reliance on ACR Appropriateness Criteria for currently available decision support tools, which may not lend themselves to helping direct nuanced decision-making for advanced imaging studies. Regardless, starting in 2017, clinical decision support will be required in ambulatory settings for radiology reimbursement of advanced imaging examinations by the Protecting Access to Medicare Act of 2014.

References

1. Smith-Bindman R, Miglioretti DL, Johnson E, et al. Use of diagnostic studies and associated radiation exposure for patients enrolled in large integrated health care systems, 1996–2010. *JAMA*. 2012;307(22):2400–2409.
2. International Atomic Energy Agency. International basic safety standards for protection against ionizing radiation and for the safety of radiation sources (Safety Series no. 115). Vienna: International Atomic Energy Agency; 1996. http://www.ilo.org/wcmsp5/groups/public/@ed_protect/@protrav/@safework/documents/publication/wcms_152685.pdf. Accessed July 28, 2015.
3. US Nuclear Regulatory Commission. NRC Regulations (10 CFR) Part 20: standards for protection against risks: subpart C, occupational dose limits. Available at: http://www.nrc.gov/reading-rm/doc-collections/cfr/part020/full-text.html. Revised February 17, 2016. Accessed July 28, 2015.
4. Preston DL, Ron E, Tokuoka S, et al. Solid cancer incidence in atomic bomb survivors: 1958–1998. *Radiat Res*. 2007;168(1):1–64.
5. Levin DC, Rao VM, Parker L, Frangos AJ, Sunshine JH. Bending the curve: the recent marked slowdown in growth of noninvasive diagnostic imaging. *AJR Am J Roentgenol*. 2011;196(1):W25–W29.
6. Hussey PS, Timbie JW, Burgette LF, Wenger NS, Nyweide DJ, Kahn KL. Appropriateness of advanced diagnostic imaging ordering before and after implementation of clinical decision support systems. *JAMA*. 2015;313(21):2181–2182.

Low-Dose Ionizing Radiation
from Medical Imaging

CHRISTOPH I. LEE

Generalization of our findings to the nonelderly adult population of the United States suggests that these procedures lead to cumulative effective doses that exceed 20 mSv per year in approximately 4 million Americans.

—FAZEL ET AL.[1]

Research Question: What is the magnitude of low-dose ionizing radiation exposure from medical imaging among the general population?

Funding: No external funding.

Years of Study: 2005–2007

Year Study Published: 2009

Study Location: Five health care markets across the United States: Arizona; Dallas; Orlando, Florida; South Florida; and Wisconsin.

Who Was Studied: Nonelderly adults ages 18–64 years continuously enrolled in a UnitedHealthcare plan during the years of study.

Who Was Excluded: Elderly patients (≥65 years) and any enrollees that did not remain alive during the study period.

How Many Patients: 952,420

Study Overview: Retrospective cohort study with use of claims data from a single large health care organization. Imaging utilization data were used to estimate cumulative effective doses.

Data Sources: All claims submitted during the study period were examined for Current Procedural Terminology codes related to imaging procedures involving ionizing radiation with exclusion of procedures delivered for therapeutic purposes. All procedures were categorized based on imaging technique and anatomic area of focus. Estimates of typical effective doses for each imaging procedure were obtained from the literature.

Endpoints: Imaging procedure frequencies and population-based rates of medical imaging-related radiation exposure according to the following cumulative effective dose categories: low (≤3 mSv/year, the natural background level of radiation in the United states[2]), moderate (>3–20 mSv per year, the upper limit for occupational exposure for at-risk workers averaged over 5 years[3]), high (>20–50 mSv, the upper limit for occupational exposure for at-risk workers in any given year[3]), or very high (>50 mSv/year).

RESULTS

- A total of 3,442,111 imaging procedures associated with radiation exposure were performed among 68.8% (655,613/952,420) of enrollees during the 3-year study period, with a mean of 1.2 ± 1.8 procedures per person per year.
- The mean cumulative effective dose (± SD) per enrollee per year was 2.4 ± 6.0 mSv with a wide distribution (median effective dose of 0.1 mSv/enrollee/year; interquartile range, 0.0–1.7).
- Overall, 193.8 enrollees per 1,000 per year incurred moderate effective doses, 18.6 enrollees per 1,000 per year incurred high effective doses, and 1.9 enrollees per 1,000 per year incurred very high effective doses. Each of these rates rose with age (see Table 50.1).
- CT and nuclear medicine imaging accounted for 21.0% of all imaging procedures, but 75.4% of the cumulative effective dose.
- Chest imaging procedures accounted for 45.2% of the total effective dose.

- The majority of the total effective dose (81.8%) was administered in the outpatient setting, most often in physicians' offices.

Table 50.1. RATES OF EXPOSURE TO VARYING ANNUAL EFFECTIVE DOSES FROM MEDICAL IMAGING

Characteristic	Low Dose (≤3 mSv/yr)	Moderate Dose (>3–20 mSv/yr)	High Dose (>20–50 mSv/yr)	Very High Dose (>50 mSv/yr)
		Number/1,000 Enrollees		
All patients	785.7	193.8	18.6	1.9
Sex				
Male	796.0	182.8	19.4	1.8
Female	776.4	203.8	17.9	1.9
Age (Years)				
18–34	895.9	98.7	4.9	0.5
35–39	845.5	145.2	8.5	0.8
40–44	809.3	177.5	12.0	1.2
45–49	770.4	209.2	18.4	2.0
50–54	719.0	252.2	26.2	2.7
55–59	668.4	289.7	38.4	3.5
60–64	598.2	343.4	52.7	5.7

mSv/yr = millisieverts per year.

Criticisms and Limitations: Claims data analysis did not allow for evaluation of imaging appropriateness. Exposure rates may have been underestimated since certain procedures involving ionizing radiation (e.g., dental radiographs) are not captured by claims data. Estimates of effective dose, rather than actual effective doses, were used. The patient population was restricted to insured patients in 5 health care markets.

Other Relevant Studies and Information:

- Approaches for justifying clinical need and optimizing use of advanced imaging will likely require health care providers to recognize and inform patients about potential risks of radiation; however, many patients and providers may not be aware that CT is associated with an increased risk of cancer.[4]
- A publicly available radiation risk calculator, based on the linear no-threshold model, is available online that provides estimates of lifetime risk of developing cancer from exposure ionizing radiation based on organ-specific doses and an individual's characteristics.[5]

- Some have advocated for use of institutional electronic medical records that can create patient radiation dose histories, with the assistance of automated dose capturing technologies, that can help track a patient's cumulative radiation exposure.[6,7]
- One potential harm of individual radiation dose histories, which are increasingly becoming a part of patients' medical records, is the sunk-cost bias—the notion that a physician may inappropriately incorporate prior exposure history in an individual patient's current risk-benefit assessment for advanced imaging.[8]

Summary and Implications: A substantial proportion of the nonelderly US population is exposed to medium to very high annual effective doses from medical imaging procedures. Strategies ensuring the appropriate use of medical imaging associated with ionizing radiation should be developed and adopted widely.

CLINICAL CASE: CUMULATIVE RADIATION EXPOSURE

Case History:
A 29-year-old male presents to the emergency department with fever, nausea, and abdominal pain that has now localized to his right lower quadrant. He has a personal history of testicular cancer that was cured 1 year ago, but for which he underwent innumerable CT scans. His institutional electronic medical record places his cumulative radiation exposure at 220 mSv. Targeted abdominal ultrasound is equivocal without identification of the appendix. How should you weigh the patient's cumulative radiation exposure and the ordering of an abdominal CT scan?

Suggested Answer:
Tracking cumulative radiation exposure can be useful in eliminating duplicate, unnecessary advanced imaging that imparts ionizing radiation. However, physicians should not fall prey to the sunk-cost bias, where prior irrevocable exposure unduly influences the calculation of future benefits and harms.[7] In this case, the fact that this patient has been exposed to a large amount of ionizing radiation in the past should not sway you from ordering a clinically indicated imaging examination. The prior radiation exposure is a sunk cost that cannot be ameliorated by not ordering this necessary abdominal CT scan for a new clinical indication.

References

1. Fazel R, Krumholz HM, Wang Y, et al. Exposure to low-dose ionizing radiation from medical imaging procedures. *N Engl J Med.* 2009;361(9):849–857.
2. Brenner DJ, Doll R, Goodhead DT, et al. Cancer risks attributable to low doses of ionizing radiation: assessing what we really know. *Proc Natl Acad Sci USA.* 2003;100:13761–13766.
3. The 2007 recommendations of the International Commission on Radiological Protection: ICRP publication 103. *Ann ICRP.* 2007;37(2–4):1–332.
4. Lee CI, Haims AH, Monico EP, Brink JA, Forman HP. Diagnostic CT scans: assessment of patient, physician, and radiologist awareness of radiation dose and possible risks. *Radiology.* 2004;231(2):393–398.
5. National Cancer Institute. Radiation Risk Assessment Tool (RadRAT). https://irep.nci.nih.gov/radrat. Accessed August 3, 2015.
6 Durand DJ. A rational approach to the clinical use of cumulative effective dose estimates. *AJR Am J Roentgenol.* 2011;197(1):160–162.
7. Raff GL, Chinnaiyan KM, Share DA, et al. Radiation dose from cardiac computed tomography before and after implementation of radiation dose-reduction techniques. *JAMA.* 2009;301(22):2340–2348.
8. Eisenberg JD, Harvey HB, Moore DA, Gazelle GS, Pandharipande PV. Falling prey to the sunk cost bias: a potential harm of patient radiation dose histories. *Radiology.* 2012;263(3):626–628.

Index

References to figures, tables, boxes and footnotes are denoted by an italicized *f*, *t*, *b* and *n*